WALL PILATES FOR MENOPAUSE WOMEN

*28-Day Challenge Over 50 illustrated,
step-by-step exercises for beginners and seniors
to achieve flexibility and balance*

Paul D Nesmith.

Disclaimer

Table of Contents

5.Wall assisted Mountain Climber.

6.Wall assisted Russian twist.

7.Wall assisted Bicycle crunches.

8.Wall plie squat.

9.Wall assisted standing forward bend.

10.Wall assisted warrior 111 pose.

11.Wall assisted Chair Pose.

12.Wall assisted Single deadlift.

13.Wall assisted side leg raises.

14.Wall assisted table top.

15.Wall assisted supine toe taps.

16.Wall assisted glute Bridge.

17.Wall assisted Forearm plank.

18.Wall assisted dead bug.

19.Wall assisted scissors kick.

20.Wall assisted oblique V ups.

21.Wall assisted hip hinge.

22.Wall assisted clamshells.

23.Wall assisted donkey kicks.

24.Wall assisted side lunges.

25.Wall assisted reverse lunges.

26.Wall assisted curtsy lunges.

27.Wall assisted standing hip abduction.

28.Wall assisted standing knee raises.

29.Wall assisted standing hamstring curls.

30.Wall assisted standing calf raises.

31.Wall assisted squat with medicine ball.

32.Wall assisted rotational squat.

33.Wall assisted tuck jumps.

Techniques for reducing anxiety & improving mental well-being.

Chapter7: Advance Wall Pilates for Progression.

1.Wall plank.

2.Wall push ups:

3.Wall squat.

4.Wall assisted leg Squat.

5.Wall Sit.

6.Wall assisted pike push ups.

7.Wall assisted L sit.

8.Wall Bridge.

9.Wall Assisted Handstand.

10.Wall Assisted Side plank.

Chapter8: Cool Down & Relaxation.

Importance of post workout cool down for Menopausal Women.

Conclusion

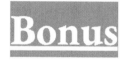

How to use this book.

1. Determine your needs: As a reader, consider your personal needs and objectives with the use of exercise to manage menopausal symptoms. It would be easier for you to concentrate on the relevant chapters and tasks in the book if you are aware of your unique issues.

2. Go over the opening: Start by reading the introduction to the book, which offers insightful information about the advantages of wall Pilates for women going through menopause. The author's background, experiences, and the rationale for this strategy's efficacy may also be covered in this part.

3. Examine the content: The book is probably broken up into parts or chapters that address various facets of Pilates workouts and menopause. Spend some time reading each chapter to learn about the physiological changes that occur during menopause and the Pilates workouts that are designed to target those changes.

4. Pay attention to the instructions: Detailed instructions for completing particular activities should be included in each chapter. Pay special attention to the breathing exercises, appropriate form, and adjustments for different levels of fitness as you properly follow these directions. It's crucial to perform the exercises as directed in a safe and individualized manner.

5. Establish a routine: Wall Pilates exercises can help you stay physically and mentally strong during menopause, which can present a number of obstacles. Make your own workout schedule using the book as a guide, taking into account your preferences, energy level, and time constraints.

6. Monitor your progress: To keep track of your advancement throughout the book, think about maintaining a journal or log. Keep track of any enhancements in mood, strength, flexibility, balance, or lessening menopausal symptoms. In this manner, you may keep an eye on your progress and draw inspiration from the improvements you see.

7. If necessary, seek expert advice: Even though the book can offer helpful exercises and information, it's always a good idea to speak with a licensed Pilates instructor or other healthcare provider, particularly if you have any concerns or pre-existing medical conditions.

8. Participate in a community: Seek out online forums, communities, or social media pages devoted to wall Pilates or menopause fitness. Talk about your experiences, pose inquiries, and offer assistance to those on a comparable path. Making connections with people can give you a sense of community and extra incentive.

Recall that while the book can serve as a helpful tool, your dedication, perseverance, and ability to modify the exercises to meet your own needs will ultimately determine your level of success. Savor the experience of using wall Pilates to enhance your general health and control menopausal symptoms!

Introduction

If you are experiencing weakness in your pelvic floor muscles, Pilates for menopause can help you live a more comfortable life.

Sneezing and having to make hurried runs to the bathroom in a panic, never knowing if you'll make it in time, may be rather annoying.

If this describes you, Pilates can help strengthen your lower back. Paul D. Nesmith, a physiotherapist and fitness instructor, is here to provide you with comprehensive guidance so you can give the absorbent pads a try. Discover all the information you require about Pilates during menopause by continuing to read.

Lifestyle Changes Work for My Wife Anabelle D Nesmith.

Even though I was married to a medical expert, I had some confusion when my own perimenopause began.

Not only was there no visible heat flush, but my sleep was severely disrupted. Fatigue soon arrived, along with a grumpy attitude. I was taking wine to calm myself and coffee to get me going.

It didn't seem like a smart long-term plan, and it wasn't me at all. My hubby concurred! Both my mood and my sleep pattern have much improved with HRT, my family informs me.

I've also adopted a healthier diet. Because I'm only 5'1", I don't have much space to conceal more weight, so I tackled menopause weight gain early on.

Once a lifelong lover of carbohydrates, I now surprise even myself by scarfing down a salad at lunch. I don't feel hungry or drowsy during the afternoon as a result.

Thinking back and understanding the research, it seems likely that maintaining an active lifestyle and eating a healthy food is preventing the physical signs of menopause.

I do observe that when I take a break from my regular, healthier routines, such wall Pilates, my mood suffers.

Paul D. Nesmith is my hero, and I have to admit that by following all of his advice, I have personally lived a happy and healthy life.

Introducing wall pilates, an empowering and life-changing workout regimen created especially for women going through menopause.

A woman's physical health, emotional stability, and general quality of life can all be impacted by the normal and important transitional phase known as menopause, which is characterized by hormonal shifts.

But with wall pilates, women can take back control, find their balance, and confidently develop their bodies.

We will examine the advantages of wall pilates for menopausal women in this in-depth tutorial, as well as the particular difficulties that women encounter at this time and how this workout method might help.

This resource intends to educate and empower you to embrace wall pilates as a potent tool in your health and wellness path, regardless of whether you are going through or have already entered menopause.

Why Pilates?

Pilates is a well-known form of exercise that emphasizes the mind-body connection, flexibility, and strength of the core.

It adds another level to the practice and provides menopausal women who are trying to restore their physical strength with stability, alignment, and a challenge when combined with the supportive factor of a wall.

The Benefits of Wall Pilates for Menopausal Women:

1.Regaining Balance: Menopause can lead to a number of physical changes, such as a decrease in muscle tone, bone density, and general balance.

Women can improve their stability, balance, and coordination in a safe atmosphere with wall pilates, which lowers their chance of accidents and falls.

2. Strengthening the Core: During menopause, back pain, poor posture, and spine support are major issues that the core—the body's powerhouse—must address. By focusing on the core muscles, wall pilates helps to stabilize and strengthen the entire body.

3. Improving Flexibility: During the menopause, hormonal fluctuations can cause joint stiffness and a loss in flexibility. Wall pilates encourages flexibility and relieves joint and muscle pain by using controlled motions, moderate stretches, and lengthening techniques.

4. *Encouraging Mental Health:* Emotional difficulties including mood swings, anxiety, and tension can be brought on by menopause.

Wall pilates' mindful methodology promotes emotional balance and general well-being by encouraging deep breathing, mental attention, and relaxation.

5. *Boosting Body Confidence:* Because of changes in weight distribution or physical appearance, menopause frequently causes issues with body image.

With self-acceptance, strength, and confidence, wall pilates helps women embrace their changing bodies. It also promotes a good body-mind connection.

Adding Wall Pilates to Your Menopause Experience:

You may be wondering how to begin now that you have a peek of the incredible advantages wall pilates offers for menopausal ladies.

We will walk you through basic exercises, adaptations for varying levels of fitness, and professional advice for a successful wall pilates practice throughout our course.

Take charge of your strength, balance, and overall well-being by starting this empowering wall pilates adventure for menopausal women.

Come explore the life-changing potential of this distinctive workout method and learn how wall pilates can help you face menopause with grace and vigor. Let's get started!

Chapter1:Understanding Menopause and Its Effects.

Definition & Stages of menopause

The end of a woman's reproductive years is marked by the natural biological process known as menopause.

It marks a crucial turning point in a woman's life and is accompanied by a number of emotional, hormonal, and physical changes.

To assist readers comprehend and negotiate this crucial time in a woman's life, we will examine the meaning of menopause and its various stages in this article. We will also offer factual, educational, and interactive material.

I. Definition of Menopause

The menstrual cycle permanently stops as a result of the ovarian function naturally declining, which is known as the menopause. Usually, a diagnosis is made following twelve months without a menstrual cycle. Two important hormones involved in the reproductive cycle, progesterone and estrogen, are gradually produced less frequently, which leads to this physiological shift.

Perimenopause

The menopausal transition, or perimenopause, is the period of time before menopause. Though some women may experience it as early as their mid-30s, it typically begins in their 40s. Hormone levels change throughout this time, and irregular menstrual cycles are possible. Hot flashes, nocturnal sweats, mood swings, sleep issues, dry vagina, and changes in libido are typical perimenopausal symptoms. This period can vary from person to person but usually lasts for several years.

Menopause

When a woman has missed her monthly cycle for twelve months in a row, she enters menopause. It typically affects people between the ages of 45 and 55, with 51 being the average age. At this point, the ovaries stop producing eggs and produce much less hormone. It is possible for perimenopausal symptoms to persist or worsen during menopause. Women may also have changes in their urine, weight gain, dry skin, and thinning hair in addition to the previously listed symptoms.

Postmenopause

The time after menopause is referred to as the postmenopause. While some women continue to endure symptoms for years, most menopausal symptoms generally lessen throughout this time. Lower hormone levels cause some health issues including osteoporosis and cardiovascular disease to become more likely. During postmenopause, maintaining general health becomes increasingly dependent on regular health exams and a balanced lifestyle.

Managing Menopausal Symptoms

Enhancing quality of life and managing menopausal symptoms can be done in a number of ways. It can be advantageous to make lifestyle adjustments including getting enough sleep, managing stress, eating a balanced diet, and exercising frequently. Hormone replacement treatment (HRT) and nonhormonal medicines can also be used to treat some symptoms. While there is conflicting scientific evidence about the efficacy of alternative therapies like acupuncture and herbal remedies, some women also use them.

Emotional and Psychological Impact

Menopause causes emotional and psychological shifts in addition to physical ones. During this time, mood swings, anxiety, irritability, and depression are common in women. A optimistic outlook, asking for help from family or medical professionals, and acknowledging and communicating these emotions can all be very helpful in overcoming the emotional challenges of menopause.

Maintaining Bone and Heart Health

Women who have gone through menopause are more likely to suffer osteoporosis and cardiovascular illnesses. Taking action to preserve heart and bone health is imperative. These risks can be decreased by engaging in regular exercise, getting enough calcium and vitamin D, abstaining from smoking and excessive alcohol use, and getting regular health examinations.

Common Symptoms Challenges Faced by Menopausal Women

We will look at some of the typical menopausal symptoms and difficulties in this book.

1. Hot flashes: Among the most well-known signs and symptoms of menopause, hot flashes are experienced by women. Sweating, flushing, and an elevated heart rate might be brought on by these abrupt and strong heat sensations.

Certain foods, alcohol, caffeine, stress, and temperature fluctuations can all cause hot flashes.

Hormone replacement treatment, additional drugs, and lifestyle changes like utilizing fans and lighter clothing can all be helpful in controlling hot flashes.

2. Night sweats: Excessive sweating while you sleep is the same as hot flashes. These episodes might cause weariness and irritability in women by upsetting their sleep patterns.

Avoiding caffeine and spicy meals right before bed, wearing permeable bedding, sleeping in a cool atmosphere, and engaging in relaxation exercises are some strategies for controlling night sweats.

3. Mood swings: Hormonal changes brought on by menopause can cause irritation, anxiety, melancholy, and mood swings.

A woman's everyday life and relationships may be impacted by these emotional shifts, which can range in intensity.

Mood-related problems can be lessened by seeking support through counseling, exercising frequently, learning stress-reduction strategies, and leading a healthy lifestyle.

4. Sleep disturbances: Women may find it more difficult to get asleep or stay asleep through the night as a result of the regular changes in sleep patterns brought on by menopause.

Disturbances in sleep may be a factor in daytime tiredness, agitation, and difficulty focusing. You may enhance the quality of your sleep by establishing a regular sleep schedule, making your bedroom comfortable, minimizing naps during the day, and avoiding stimulating activities just before bed.

5. Vaginal dryness: The thinning of the vaginal tissues and vaginal dryness can be caused by the menopause's declining estrogen levels.

This may result in pain during sexual activity, discomfort, and a higher risk of UTIs.

Vaginal dryness can be controlled with over-the-counter lubricants, moisturizers, and hormone replacement medication that has been prescribed by a medical professional.

6. Decreased libido: Another effect of fluctuating hormone levels is a reduction in libido, or the desire for sexual activity.

Women going through menopause may notice changes in their ability to conceive, such as decreased arousal and trouble getting an orgasm.

Having an honest conversation with a spouse, getting support from a medical professional, and trying out new enjoyable hobbies can all help deal with these issues.

7. Concerns about bone health: Women are more vulnerable to osteoporosis and bone loss after menopause due to a decrease in estrogen levels.

Because of this disorder, bones become weaker and are more likely to break. Osteoporosis can be prevented or managed by following a nutritious diet high in calcium and vitamin D, exercising with weights, and talking with a healthcare professional about bone health drugs.

8. Changes in metabolism and weight gain: Because menopause tends to lower metabolic rates, it might cause weight gain, especially around the abdomen.

You may control weight growth and preserve general health by eating a balanced diet, exercising frequently, and doing strength training activities.

9. Memory and cognitive changes: Memory, focus, and cognitive function can be problematic for certain women going through menopause.

These adjustments might affect day-to-day tasks and be annoying. Managing cognitive problems can be facilitated by getting support from healthcare specialists, participating in mentally challenging activities, and keeping a healthy lifestyle.

10. Risks to heart health: Although estrogen helps to protect the heart, its decrease after menopause raises the possibility of cardiovascular illnesses.

Heart disease risk can be decreased by leading a heart-healthy lifestyle, which includes quitting smoking, managing stress, eating a balanced diet, and getting regular exercise.

It is significant to remember that not every woman going through menopause has the same problems or symptoms; some may have very minimal or nonexistent symptoms.

Since every woman's experience with menopause is different, consulting with medical specialists can help give tailored solutions for symptom management and general wellbeing during this phase of life.

Women normally go through the menopause, a normal biological process, between the ages of 45 and 55.

Menstrual periods finish at this point because the ovaries stop releasing eggs and produce less hormones. Menopause is a natural stage of a woman's life, but it can also have a variety of negative effects on her general health.

We will look at some of the typical menopausal symptoms and difficulties in this book

1. Hot flashes: Among the most well-known signs and symptoms of menopause, hot flashes are experienced by women. Sweating, flushing, and an elevated heart rate might be brought on by these abrupt and strong heat sensations.

Certain foods, alcohol, caffeine, stress, and temperature fluctuations can all cause hot flashes.

Hormone replacement treatment, additional drugs, and lifestyle changes like utilizing fans and lighter clothing can all be helpful in controlling hot flashes.

2. Night sweats: Excessive sweating while you sleep is the same as hot flashes. These episodes might cause weariness and irritability in women by upsetting their sleep patterns.

Avoiding caffeine and spicy meals right before bed, wearing permeable bedding, sleeping in a cool atmosphere, and engaging in relaxation exercises are some strategies for controlling night sweats.

3. Mood swings: Hormonal changes brought on by menopause can cause irritation, anxiety, melancholy, and mood swings.

A woman's everyday life and relationships may be impacted by these emotional shifts, which can range in intensity.

Mood-related problems can be lessened by seeking support through counseling, exercising frequently, learning stress-reduction strategies, and leading a healthy lifestyle.

4. Sleep disturbances: Women may find it more difficult to get asleep or stay asleep through the night as a result of the regular changes in sleep patterns brought on by menopause.

Disturbances in sleep may be a factor in daytime tiredness, agitation, and difficulty focusing.

You may enhance the quality of your sleep by establishing a regular sleep schedule, making your bedroom comfortable, minimizing naps during the day, and avoiding stimulating activities just before bed.

5. Vaginal dryness: The thinning of the vaginal tissues and vaginal dryness can be caused by the menopause's declining estrogen levels.

This may result in pain during sexual activity, discomfort, and a higher risk of UTIs.

Vaginal dryness can be controlled with over-the-counter lubricants, moisturizers, and hormone replacement medication that has been prescribed by a medical professional.

6. Decreased libido: Another effect of fluctuating hormone levels is a reduction in libido, or the desire for sexual activity.

Women going through menopause may notice changes in their ability to conceive, such as decreased arousal and trouble getting an orgasm.

Having an honest conversation with a spouse, getting support from a medical professional, and trying out new enjoyable hobbies can all help deal with these issues.

7. Concerns about bone health: Women are more vulnerable to osteoporosis and bone loss after menopause due to a decrease in estrogen levels.

Because of this disorder, bones become weaker and are more likely to break. Osteoporosis can be prevented or managed by following a nutritious diet high in calcium and vitamin D, exercising with weights, and talking with a healthcare professional about bone health drugs.

8. Changes in metabolism and weight gain: Because menopause tends to lower metabolic rates, it might cause weight gain, especially around the abdomen.

You may control weight growth and preserve general health by eating a balanced diet, exercising frequently, and doing strength training activities.

9. Memory and cognitive changes: Memory, focus, and cognitive function can be problematic for certain women going through menopause.

These adjustments might affect day-to-day tasks and be annoying.

Managing cognitive problems can be facilitated by getting support from healthcare specialists, participating in mentally challenging activities, and keeping a healthy lifestyle.

10. Risks to heart health: Although estrogen helps to protect the heart, its decrease after menopause raises the possibility of cardiovascular illnesses.

Heart disease risk can be decreased by leading a heart-healthy lifestyle, which includes quitting smoking, managing stress, eating a balanced diet, and getting regular exercise.

It is significant to remember that not every woman going through menopause has the same problems or symptoms; some may have very minimal or nonexistent symptoms. Since every woman's experience with menopause is different, consulting with medical specialists can help give tailored solutions for symptom management and general wellbeing during this phase of life.

Hormonal Changes & Their Impacts on the Body & Mind

The decrease in estrogen levels during menopause is one of the main hormonal changes that take place.

In addition to lowering cholesterol levels, preserving bone density, and promoting general cardiovascular health, estrogen is the hormone that controls the menstrual cycle.

Women may have symptoms like vaginal dryness, night sweats, and hot flashes when their estrogen levels drop.

Additionally affecting bone health and raising the risk of osteoporosis is the decrease in estrogen.

A deficiency in estrogen can weaken bones and increase the risk of fractures. This highlights how crucial it is to keep up a healthy lifestyle throughout menopause, which includes frequent exercise and a well-balanced diet high in calcium and vitamin D.

Another hormone that decreases with menopause is progesterone, which is also important for pregnancy and the menstrual cycle.

Mood swings and irregular periods may result from its decline. Since progesterone is also known to have soothing effects, a decrease in it may be a factor in the rise in irritation and anxiety.

The physical and mental health of a woman may be directly impacted by these hormonal fluctuations.

Apart from the physiological manifestations previously discussed, menopause can also impact sleep cycles, resulting in challenges in initiating and maintaining sleep throughout the night.

Throughout the day, this may cause weariness, low energy, and trouble concentrating.

Hormone fluctuations can also impact memory and cognitive performance. Forgetting things or having trouble multitasking are common symptoms among women, which are commonly called "brain fog."

 It is evident that hormone changes can affect mental functions, even though the precise relationship between these changes and cognitive performance is still being investigated.

A woman's emotional condition can be significantly impacted by menopause as well. During this period, mood swings, depression, and elevated anxiety are typical.

The brain's neurotransmitters, which include dopamine and serotonin and are in charge of mood regulation, are intricately regulated by hormones. These neurotransmitters can be upset by imbalances in hormones, which can cause mood disorders.

It is noteworthy that certain ladies may not encounter these symptoms to the same extent or perhaps at all.

A woman's menopausal experience can be influenced by a number of factors, including her lifestyle, genetics, and general health.

Hormone replacement treatment (HRT) may provide relief for certain women; alternate methods such as herbal supplements or lifestyle modifications may be explored by others.

Chapter2: Introduction to Wall Pilates

What is Wall Pilates & How it Benefits Menopausal Women.

For women going through menopause, wall Pilates is a novel and very beneficial kind of exercise.

Wall Pilates integrates the foundations of classical Pilates with the stability and support offered by the wall. It was created to include the use of a wall as a prop.

This novel method assists women going through menopause in maintaining general fitness, strengthening their core, increasing their flexibility, and adjusting to the mental and physical changes that come with going through menopause.

Many women suffer from a reduction in muscle mass, an increase in joint stiffness, and a decrease in bone density throughout menopause.

An elevated risk of osteoporosis and other musculoskeletal problems may result from these alterations.

Wall Pilates is a low-impact, high-impact exercise program that prevents muscle loss, enhances bone density, and increases joint mobility.

Strengthening and stabilizing the core is one of the main advantages of Wall Pilates for women going through menopause.

Women may see a loss in muscle mass following menopause, particularly in the abdominal area, when their estrogen levels drop.

A strong core is essential for supporting good posture, the health of the spine, and the prevention of lower back discomfort.

Because Wall Pilates uses the wall to provide additional support and stability, it is especially helpful for women who may struggle with balance or feel insecure in their movements.

Menopausal women can strengthen their entire body and engage their core muscles while feeling comfortable and supported by combining mat work movements like leg circles, pelvic curls, and abdominal curls with the use of the wall as a prop.

Wall Pilates improves joint mobility and flexibility in addition to core strength.

When stretches are done against a wall, they aid to lengthen muscles, expand their range of motion, and strengthen joints.

Women going through menopause, whose hormones may cause joint stiffness, can particularly benefit from this.

Frequent Wall Pilates practice can help with these symptoms, increase range of motion, and lower the chance of injury.

Furthermore, mood swings, anxiety, and depression are among the emotional changes that menopause frequently brings about.

Exercise, particularly Wall Pilates, has been demonstrated to improve mood by causing the body's endorphins—natural feel-good chemicals—to be released.

Regular Wall Pilates practice can improve general well-being, improve mood, and assist menopausal women handle stress.

Every woman experiences menopause differently, so it's vital to remember that. Before beginning any new fitness regimen, it's best to speak with a healthcare provider.

A trained Pilates instructor with experience working with menopausal women can also offer individualized support and guarantee that exercises are done correctly.

To sum up, wall Pilates has many advantages for women going through menopause, such as increased flexibility, stronger core, and better joint mobility.

This exercise technique is ideal for ladies going through this transitional phase of changes in confidence or balance since it uses the wall as a prop to provide extra support and stability.

Frequent wall Pilates practice can improve general fitness, support a healthier and more active lifestyle, and assist handle the mental and physical changes related to menopause.

The Unique Advantages of Using a Wall for Exercises.

Fitness aficionados find that using a wall for training has several special benefits that make it a useful and efficient tool.

Add wall workouts to your regimen for a variety of mental and physical advantages, regardless of your level of experience or skill.

We will go over the many benefits of using a wall for exercises in this engaging and instructional guide, along with providing accurate information to help you get the most of it.

1. Stability and Safety: The stability a wall offers during exercises is one of the main benefits of employing one.

Walls provide a stable platform for a variety of actions since they are strong and dependable.

This stability is especially helpful for people who have trouble maintaining their balance or who need additional assistance when working out.

In addition, walls can act as a safety net, reducing the chance of damage and preventing falls, which makes them an invaluable resource for individuals of all fitness levels.

2. Versatility: There is nothing like the wall for versatility. It can be used for a variety of exercises that focus on distinct muscle groups and fitness objectives.

Depending on your goals, you can modify the wall to concentrate on strength, flexibility, or stability.

The options are unlimited, ranging from basic wall sits and handstands to more difficult exercises like wall push-ups and aided inversions.

This makes it possible for athletes of all skill levels to keep pushing themselves and grow in their quest for fitness.

3. Targeted Muscle Engagement: Adding a wall to your workouts gives you an additional layer of resistance.

You can use more muscles and increase the intensity of the workout by leaning or pushing against the wall. Muscle areas including the deltoids, quadriceps, hamstrings, and core can all be successfully worked out using wall workouts.

Wall squats, for instance, are a great technique to build leg strength, and wall push-ups work the triceps, shoulders, and chest.

You may maximize muscle engagement and increase the efficacy of your workouts by using a wall.

4. Postural Alignment: One helpful aid for better posture is the wall. Prolonged sitting causes bad posture in many people, which can result in a number of health problems.

You can actively focus on correcting postural imbalances, strengthening the muscles that maintain good posture, and eventually minimizing pain and discomfort by adopting wall-based exercises like wall stretches and wall angels.

5. Greater Flexibility: Often overlooked, flexibility is an essential component of fitness. Stretching exercises and improving flexibility can both benefit from using the wall.

You can safely increase the depth of your stretches and enhance your range of motion by using the wall as support.

For those who are trying to achieve splits, backbends, or other advanced stretching poses, this is especially helpful.

6. Mental Concentration and Mindfulness:

Exercise benefits our mental health in addition to its physical benefits.

The additional stability provided by working against a wall enhances the mind-muscle connection by enabling you to concentrate on the specific muscle groups you are working.

Being more mindful as a result of your heightened awareness will enable you to work out fully and in the present moment.

Stress levels can be lowered and therapeutic benefits can also result from the calming effect of concentrating on the movement against the wall.

In conclusion, there are a variety of distinct benefits to performing workouts against a wall.

The wall offers a strong basis to enhance your workouts, from stability and safety to variety and focused muscle engagement. Its advantages go beyond just physical enhancements; they also include improved mental clarity, greater flexibility, and improved posture alignment. Including wall workouts in your training regimen can be a beneficial way to improve your general health.

So, make the most of this adaptable tool and discover all of the opportunities it presents to advance your fitness path.

Importance of Proper Alignment & Safety precautions.

In order to enhance the efficiency of any type of exercise, proper alignment is essential since it creates a strong basis for movement.

Because menopause involves significant changes in the body's structure and muscular tone, it is even more crucial for women to maintain good alignment.

The body must be positioned correctly to target the targeted muscles and avoid unneeded strain or injury.

When performing wall Pilates, bear in mind the following important alignment principles:

1. Spine alignment: To begin, stand facing the wall with your back to it, making sure your head, shoulders, and hips are in contact with it. By keeping the spine in a neutral position, this lessens strain on the vertebrae and encourages proper posture.

2. Shoulder alignment: Pull your shoulders back and down a little while relaxing them away from your ears. During exercises, this position supports the upper body and optimizes shoulder stability.

3. Core engagement: Pull your navel gently toward your spine to activate your core muscles. By engaging the deep abdominal muscles, this supports proper posture, protects the lower back, and offers stability.

4. Hip alignment: To keep your balance at its best, line up your hips with your shoulders and feet. Steer clear of shifting the pelvis forward or backward as this can cause tension on the hips or lower back.

5. Knee and ankle alignment: Make sure your knees track in line with your second toe and that your weight is evenly distributed across your feet when you undertake workouts that require you to bend your knees. By doing this, the lower body's alignment is maintained and the knee joints are safeguarded.

During wall Pilates workouts, safety measures should be considered in addition to alignment. Safety should always come first since menopausal women may have changes in their joint and bone health. The following are some crucial safety precautions to remember:

1. Warm-up: To improve blood flow, warm up the muscles, and get the body ready for exercise, start each session with a little warm-up.

2. Gradual progression: Begin with simple workouts and work your way up to more difficult or intense ones over time. Steer clear of overexerting oneself or attempting complex moves without adequate training and supervision.

3. Pay attention to your body: Throughout each activity, be mindful of your feelings. Adjust the movement or get professional help if something hurts or feels unpleasant. Recognize your body's limitations and refrain from overdoing it.

4. Appropriate footwear: Select stable, sturdy footwear for wall Pilates routines. This lessens the chance of strain or injury to the ankles, foot, and joints.

5. Breath control: Pay close attention to keeping your breathing steady and under control as you perform the exercises. Inhaling and exhaling deeply helps to improve focus, relax the body, and oxygenate the muscles.

Menopausal women can work out safely and effectively with a wall Pilates practice that incorporates these alignment concepts and safety considerations.

Before beginning any new fitness program, you should, however, always get advice from a medical expert or a certified Pilates instructor, particularly if you have any particular health issues or limits.

Wall Pilates, when combined with a comprehensive commitment to safety and good alignment, can give menopausal women better posture, stronger muscles, better balance, and a general sense of well-being.

These low-impact workouts help women keep their flexibility, be active, and improve their general health both during and after menopause.

Chapter3: Getting Started: Essential Equipment & Set-up

Choosing the right wall space & clearing it for exercise

In order to guarantee a successful and pleasurable workout, we will examine the elements to take into account while selecting the ideal wall space and offer helpful advice for cleaning it.

Selecting the Appropriate Wall Area

1. Evaluate Availability: Find a wall area in your house that is big enough for your workout, well-lit, and easily accessible. Think about spaces like a living room, a spare room, or even a designated spot.

2. Assess Structural sustain: Make sure the wall area you've selected is strong enough to sustain the variety of activities you intend to perform. If necessary, seek professional advice to determine the wall's load-bearing capacity.

3. Take Privacy and Surroundings into Account:

If at all possible, choose a wall location that provides seclusion and few outside distractions.

An atmosphere that is calm and concentrated can be created by drawing curtains or using a private space.

Making Room on the Wall for Exercise

1. Remove Obstacles: Get rid of any furniture, decorations, or other materials that might get in the way of your workout-related activities. Additionally, keep the floor space surrounding the wall space clutter-free.

2. Wall Protection: To minimize damage to the walls and assure safety during high-intensity workouts or exercises involving impact, think about utilizing protective mats, foam pads, or wall coverings, depending on the sort of activities you plan to perform.

3. illumination Issues: Sustaining motivation and safety both depend on adequate illumination. Place high-quality lighting fixtures next to the wall to guarantee visibility when working out. Positive effects from natural light can also be felt in the training space.

4. Arrange Exercise Equipment: Make sure your exercise equipment is organized and stored in a productive way. To keep weights, resistance bands, yoga mats, and other training supplies well-organized and conveniently accessible, use hooks, shelves, or wall-mounted racks.

In conclusion, providing menopausal women with an exercise-friendly wall space can greatly improve their general well-being during this critical stage of life.

Women can manage menopause symptoms and get the benefits of regular physical activity by adding interactive and informative aspects, clearing out clutter, and choosing the right wall space.

Make an investment to create a customized, eye-catching workout wall space that inspires and facilitates your journey toward improved health and fitness during menopause.

Recommended Props & Equipment for wall pilates.

In order to assist you attain the best results possible, we shall examine a range of wall Pilates props and equipment below.

1. Pilates Mat: The cornerstone of each Pilates exercise, including wall Pilates, is a firm and cozy Pilates mat.

It offers support and cushioning when working out against the wall, giving you a secure platform to train on.

2. Pilates Wall Unit: Also referred to as a Pilates tower, a Pilates wall unit is made specifically to be fastened to a wall and offers a variety of anchor points for springs and resistance bands.

It is a flexible piece of wall Pilates equipment that may be used for a variety of workouts, including those that need standing and lying postures.

You can push yourself to new limits because the wall unit offers support as well as resistance.

3. Resistance Bands: Resistance bands are a great supplement to Pilates exercises performed against the wall.

To target different muscle groups, they are available in a range of strengths and resistance levels.

You can target and intensify your arm, leg, and core exercises by fastening the bands to the wall unit.

4. Foam Roller: Adding a foam roller to your wall Pilates exercise creates a sense of instability and requires you to engage your core muscles in order to stay balanced.

Exercises like leg lifts and planks can be done with the foam roller pressed up against the wall to increase intensity and test your stability.

5. Stability Ball: Often referred to as an exercise ball or a Swiss ball, a stability ball is an adaptable prop that may be utilized in a variety of wall Pilates exercises.

It enhances balance, coordination, and core strength. You can use the wall to include the stability ball into exercises like plank variants, wall squats, and ball exercises that require sitting or lying down.

6. Hand Weights: You may up the resistance and intensity of your wall Pilates exercise by incorporating hand weights.

Working your upper body to the limit while using your core for stability and control is possible with exercises like shoulder presses, tricep extensions, and bicep curls against the wall.

7. Pilates Magic Circle: A common prop in classical Pilates, the Pilates Magic Circle is also known as the fitness ring.

It assists in targeting and toning particular muscular regions, such as the arms, chest, and inner and outer thighs, when used in wall Pilates routines.

When performing arm exercises against the wall or wall squats, the Magic Circle can be positioned between the arms and legs.

8. Yoga Blocks: For people with restricted flexibility, yoga blocks can offer assistance and support during wall Pilates routines.

They can be deepened in stretches, used as props to change up workouts, and improve alignment.

A yoga block pressed up against the wall can provide stability and enable appropriate adjustments.

9. Pilates Bar: A Pilates bar is a flexible prop that may be used for workouts on the floor against the wall as well as standing.

It improves muscular activation and range of motion by adding stability and resistance to your exercises. Exercises like squats, lunges, bicep curls, and rows can be performed with the bar.

10. Towel or Yoga Strap: To help with stretching and improve flexibility, wall Pilates can be performed with a towel or yoga strap.

Stretches against the wall can be made more intense and have a wider range of motion by wrapping the strap or towel around your foot and holding onto it.

Recall that adding additional props or equipment to your wall Pilates exercise should only be done after consulting with a licensed Pilates instructor or fitness expert.

They may help you with technique and make sure you're utilizing the props in a safe and efficient manner.

To sum up, wall Pilates presents a novel take on classic Pilates movements.

You can improve your wall Pilates routine and increase your strength, flexibility, and general fitness by adding props and equipment such a Pilates wall unit, resistance bands, foam roller, stability ball, hand weights, Pilates Magic Circle, yoga blocks, Pilates bar, and towels or straps. Cheers to your wall Pilates training!

Simple techniques to warm up & prepare the body

This book will walk you through a variety of easy and efficient warm-up routines designed especially for wall pilates practitioners who are menopausal.

1. Deep Breathing: To promote focus and relaxation, start your warm-up routine with deep breathing exercises. Breathe in deeply through your nose to fill your diaphragm, then completely out through your mouth to relieve any remaining tension.

To oxygenate your muscles and get your body ready for the forthcoming workout, repeat this procedure multiple times.

2. Neck and Shoulder Rolls: To relieve stress and improve range of motion in these regions, gently roll your neck and shoulders.

To increase the range of motion, start by moving your shoulders forward in a circular motion. Next, roll your shoulders backward to perform the same action again.

Next, move your neck slowly and deliberately in both directions while avoiding discomfort and being aware of any limitations.

3. Arm Circles: Spread your arms out to the sides and, while maintaining control, move your palms down to form little circles.

As you gradually enlarge the circles, strive for smooth, controlled motions. This improves posture and alignment during wall pilates movements by warming up the shoulder and upper back muscles.

4. Standing Side Stretch: Lengthen your side by reaching your right arm overhead while keeping your feet hip-width apart.

As you feel a slight stretch along your right side, slant slightly to the left. Repeat on the opposite side after holding for a short while.

In order to prepare the body for lateral movements in wall pilates, this exercise helps lengthen the torso and stimulate the side abdominal muscles.

5. Pelvic tilts: Place your feet hip-width apart and lean your back against the wall.

By using your core, you may gradually tilt your pelvis forward, which will arch your lower back, and backward, which will round it.

Move carefully, concentrating on releasing tension in your lower back and pelvis. Pelvic tilts contribute to two key elements of wall pilates exercise: strengthening the core and improving pelvic stability.

6. Wall-Supported Squats: Lean against a wall and extend your feet a little. For support, place your hands against the wall.

With your back against the wall, slowly bend your knees and lower your body into a squat position.

As you lower yourself, exhale, and as you rise back up, engage your core. The lower body muscles, such as the hamstrings, quadriceps, and glutes, are warmed up by this exercise.

7. Cat-Cow Stretch: Drop to all fours and place your knees under your hips and your wrists under your shoulders.

Take a deep breath and slowly arch your back, lowering your head and tailbone (Cow Pose). Breathe out, turn your back, and tuck your chin into your chest to assume the cat pose.

Breathe your way between these two postures, letting it direct your actions. This stretch works the core muscles and enhances spinal mobility.

In conclusion, menopausal women doing wall pilates must warm up appropriately in order to guarantee a successful and injury-free workout.

You may maximize the benefits of wall pilates and prepare your body for its demands by implementing these easy and efficient warm-up exercises.

Always pay attention to your body, acknowledge your limits, and get medical advice before starting a new fitness program. Savor the experience of wall Pilates and acknowledge its transformational potential throughout the menopause.

Chapter4: Fundamental Wall Pilates Exercises.

Core strengthening exercises using the wall as a support

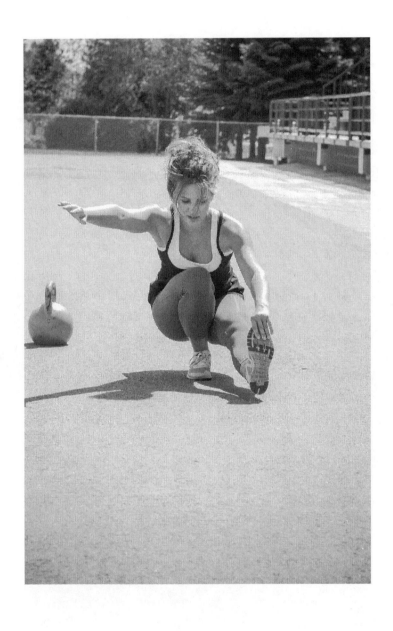

1.Wall assisted pistol squat.

Equipment needed:

- Wall or sturdy vertical surface for assistance

Time frame:

Depending on your goals and level of fitness, completing a set of repetitions will take a different amount of time. As you gain strength, progressively increase the number of repetitions from a comfortable starting point (e.g., 5–10).

Direction

1. Place your feet hip-width apart and face the wall.

2. For balance, extend your arms straight in front of you.

3. Raise your right foot off the floor while maintaining a straight leg in front of you.

4. Bend your left knee and slowly lower yourself, as though you were reclining on a chair. Keep your core active and your chest raised.

5. Lean your back slightly against the wall to support yourself as you descend.

6. Try lowering yourself as much as is comfortable until your left thigh is parallel to the floor.

7. Hold the bottom posture for a little period of time, then release your breath and push through your left heel to stand back up, making sure to activate your left glute and quadriceps.

8. Carry out the motion for the required number of times.

9. To switch sides, raise your left foot off the ground and use your right leg to complete the exercise.

Tips

Go slowly and concentrate on keeping the right form throughout the exercise.

Maintain a raised chest and a tight core to aid with stability and balance.

Try reducing the range of motion until you gain strength if you are having trouble maintaining complete stability.

When you feel more comfortable, you can try the pistol squat without any aid or use less of the wall's support to make it harder.

2.Wall assisted bird Dog.

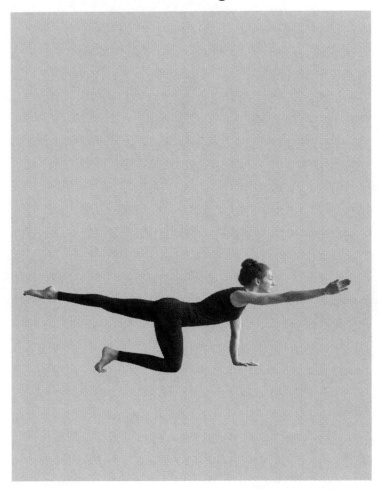

Time Frame:

This exercise can be performed for 10-15 minutes, depending on your fitness level and comfort.

Equipment/ Materials Needed:

1. Yoga mat or comfortable surface
2. Wall
3. Bed or elevated surface
4. Comfortable clothing

Direction

1. Set yourself up: Locate a free area up against the wall where you may place your yoga mat or any other cozy surface.

- Place your elevated surface, or bed, up against the wall.

- Dress comfortably so that your movements are unrestricted.

2. Warm-up: To get your body ready for exercise, begin with a light warm-up. This can involve five to ten minutes of low-impact exercise, including skipping rope or stationary jogging.

3. The "Bird Dog" Position: - Take a stand with the bed behind you and your back to the wall.

- Spread your hands shoulder-width apart on the mat or raised surface, with your fingers pointed in the direction of the bed.

- Retrace your steps with both feet, keeping your head and heels in a straight line.

- Maintain a straight back and contract your core muscles.

4. Wall-Assisted Bird Dog: - Maintain a straight posture as you slowly move your hands in the direction of the bed. An inverted "V" with your body should resemble the downward dog position in yoga.

- Extend your calves and hamstrings by pressing your palms firmly into the mat or raised surface while simultaneously pushing your heels towards the floor.

- Your hands and feet should support the same amount of your body weight. A decent stretch can be obtained by adjusting the distance between your hands and feet.

- While you hold this posture for 15 to 30 seconds, concentrate on taking deep breaths and letting go of any tension in your body.

5. Repeat: - Walk your hands slowly back towards the wall to reposition yourself in the first posture.

- After a brief period of rest, perform the Wall Assisted Bird Dog exercise again for the appropriate number of reps or amount of time.

- You can progressively increase the hold time or the number of repetitions as you gain comfort and confidence.

6. Cool Down: - To stretch and relax your muscles after your workout, use a good cool-down program.

- Target the main muscle groups used in the workout with mild stretches.

Breathe deeply and give your heart a little time to return to normal.

3.Wall assisted tricep dip.

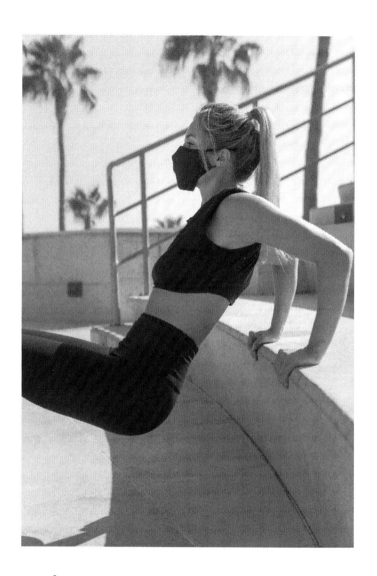

Equipment needed:

1. A sturdy wall or vertical surface.

Time frame:

Start with a comfortable number of repetitions and gradually increase as you become more comfortable and stronger. Aim for 2-3 sets of 10-15 reps.

<u>Direction</u>

1. Place your feet shoulder-width apart and stand in front of a wall or other vertical surface.

2. Spread your arms wide and press your palms flat, shoulder-height against the wall. The tips of your fingers ought to be pointing down.

3. Bend forward while maintaining your elbows close to your body and your feet firmly planted on the floor. This is where you will begin.

4. Bending your elbows while maintaining a straight back, lower your body toward the wall.

5. Keep lowering yourself until your elbows are 90 degrees or just a little bit lower.

6. Hold the bottom position for a little period of time, then straighten your arms to propel yourself back up to the beginning position.

7. To get the appropriate number of repetitions, repeat steps 4-6.

8. Throughout the exercise, be sure to contract your core muscles and keep your movement regulated.

<u>Tips</u>

Keep in mind to breathe steadily while performing the workout.

As you do the exercise, concentrate on activating your tricep muscles while maintaining shoulder stability.

Stepping closer to or further away from the wall will allow you to modify the difficulty of the workout if you find it too difficult.

Pay attention to your body's signals and cease if you feel any pain or discomfort.

4.Wall assisted Knee tuck.

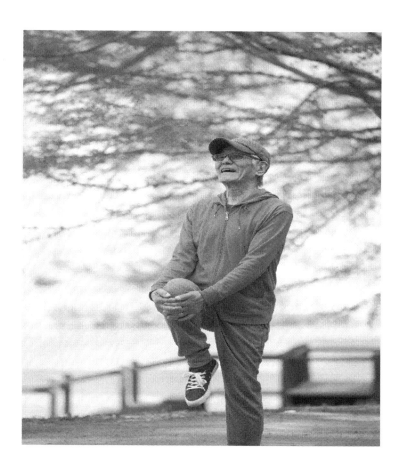

Equipment needed:

1. A sturdy wall or vertical surface.

Time frame:

The time frame for this exercise can vary depending on your fitness level and goals. It is recommended to start with 8-10 repetitions per leg and gradually increase the number of repetitions as you feel more comfortable. You can also perform multiple sets with short breaks in between for added challenge.

Direction

1. In an open area, identify a wall or other suitable vertical surface.

2. Place your feet hip-width apart and stand facing the wall.

3. Slightly bend forward and position both hands shoulder-width apart and at shoulder height on the wall.

4. Pull your belly button in the direction of your spine to activate your core muscles.

5. With your foot flexed, slowly bring one knee towards your chest. Throughout the motion, keep your spine straight.

6. At the peak of the action, pause for a little while before lowering your foot gradually back to the beginning position.

7. Switch to the other leg and repeat the motion.

8. Keep switching between the legs for however many reps or how long you want.

9. Strive for calm, controlled motions as opposed to quick ones.

10. Throughout the exercise, maintain your stability by keeping both hands firmly on the wall.

11. Pay attention to your breathing during the exercise. Take a breath during the lifting phase and release it during the lowering phase.

Always pay attention to your body's signals and quit if you feel any pain or discomfort. Before beginning any new fitness regimen, it is always a good idea to speak with a qualified fitness teacher or a member of the medical community.

5.Wall assisted Mountain Climber.

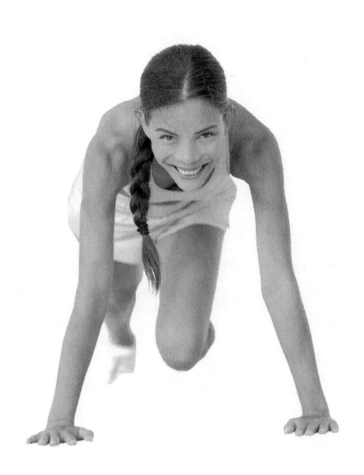

Equipment/ Material needed:

A sturdy flat wall & a comfortable workout clothes and shoes

Direction

1. Warm-up: To raise your heart rate and warm up your muscles, engage in a brief cardio workout before beginning the exercise. You can opt for exercises like walking quickly, jumping jacks, or stationary jogging.

2. Find a wall: In an area large enough to carry out the activity without any obstacles, find a stable wall or vertical surface.

3. Take a stand with your back to the wall and place your feet hip-width apart. You should be around arms' length away from the wall. The tips of your toes ought to be facing forward.

4. Assume a plank posture by placing your hands shoulder-width apart and at shoulder height on the wall. Stretch your legs backward while maintaining a straight body and your legs together. Your hands and toes should be bearing your weight.

5. Perform the mountain climber exercise: Start by activating your core. Bring your right knee as close to your chest as you can while lifting your right foot and bringing it up to your hands. Avoid lowering your head or rising your hips; instead, maintain a straight body. At the same time, raise your left knee to your chest and lower your right leg back to the beginning position. Perform this alternating motion for the required number of reps or duration, just like you would if you were climbing a mountain.

6. Maintain appropriate form: Pay attention to maintaining your back straight, your hips stable, and your core muscles activated throughout the exercise. Steer clear of bouncing or swinging too much.

7. Regulate your breathing: Take a breath as you lift each knee to your chest and release it as you stretch your leg back to the beginning.

8. Pay attention to your intensity: Modify the movement's pace and force in accordance with your degree of fitness. More experienced players can push themselves by increasing the speed and adding new variations, while beginners can start out more slowly.

9. Establish a target: Establish the target number of repetitions or time interval (e.g., 30 seconds or 1 minute) for each set. As you gain endurance and strength, gradually increase the number of repetitions or length.

10. Cool down: Once the required number of sets has been completed, carry out a cool-down exercise. Stretch your muscles for a few minutes, paying particular attention to your upper, lower, and core.

6.Wall assisted Russian twist.

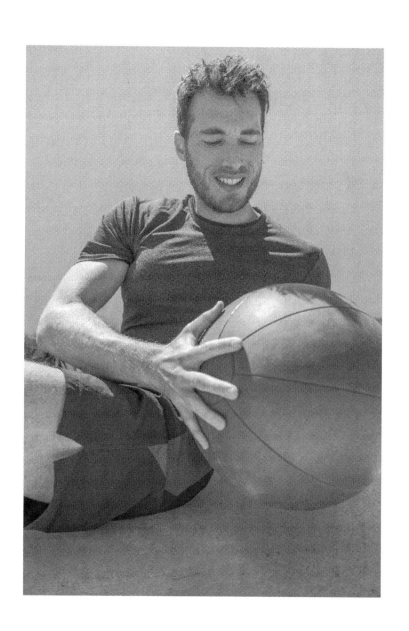

Equipment needed:

1. An exercise mat or a soft surface to sit on.

Medicine ball (optional)

Time frame:

Start with 2-3 sets of 10-12 repetitions and gradually increase as you get comfortable with the exercise.

Direction

1. Locate a spot on a wall that is free of obstructions so that you may sit comfortably with your back to the wall.

2. Lay down a cushioned surface on the ground, such as an exercise mat.

3. Place your feet flat on the ground and sit on the mat with your knees bent. Make sure your back is touching the wall.

4. Slightly recline while still keeping your body in contact with the wall. Make sure your spine is neutral and that your core is active.

5. Put your arms out in front of your chest and interlace your fingers.

6. Raise your feet a few inches above the ground. Your core muscles will be put in a difficult posture as a result.

7. Twist your body to the right while maintaining your back against the wall and your core active.

8. After a brief pause, swivel your torso to the left and take a step back to the beginning. One iteration is finished with this.

9. Alternate between the sides and do the twisting motion for the required amount of repetitions.

10. Throughout the workout, pay attention to keeping your movements smooth and under control. Steer clear of jerking or employing momentum.

11. Breathe steadily and slowly during the activity.

12. Lower your feet and take a brief break after reaching the target number of repetitions before starting new sets.

7.Wall Assisted Bicycle crunches.

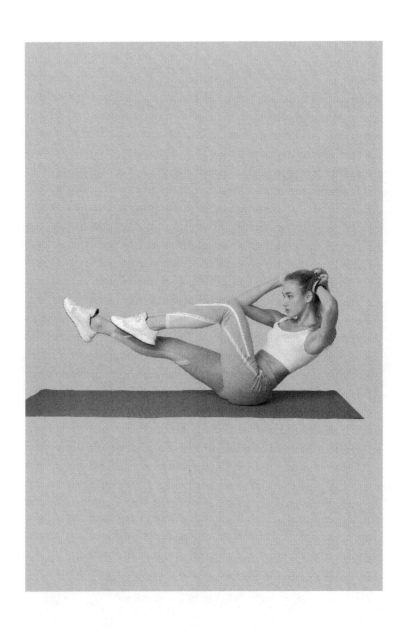

Equipment needed:

A sturdy flat wall

Time frame:

Start with 10-15 minutes and gradually increase the duration as you get comfortable with the exercise.

Direction

1. Locate a free wall space and make sure it's unobstructed.
2. Position the workout mat in front of the wall on the floor.
3. Place your back on the floor while lying down on the mat.
4. Ensure that your lower back is forced on the mat by positioning yourself near to the wall.
5. Raise your legs straight out in front of the wall.

6. With your elbows pointed outward, place your hands gently on the sides of your head.

7. Keep your elbows wide and your chin up as you lift your upper body slightly off the mat to engage your core.

8. Bring your right knee up to your chest to start the exercise.

9. Twist your upper body and bend your left elbow toward your right knee at the same time.

10. As you fully extend your left leg, straighten your right leg and maintain it off the wall.

11. At this point, twist your upper body and pull your right elbow toward your left knee as you bring your left knee closer to your chest.

12. Using your left and right knees in turn, imitate a cycling action.

13. Keep up the steady, rhythmic cycling action while keeping your composure.

14. Depending on your level of fitness, try to complete this exercise for a set amount of repetitions or for a set amount of time.

15. Lower your upper body carefully and relax your legs back to the starting position after performing the required number of repetitions or time.

16. Before you resume or end your exercise, take a few deep breaths and relax for a bit.

Always remember to use good form, use your core, and concentrate on deliberate motions as opposed to rapidity. Pay attention to your body's signals and quit if you feel any pain or discomfort. As usual, prior to beginning any new fitness program, get medical advice.

8.Wall Plie Squat.

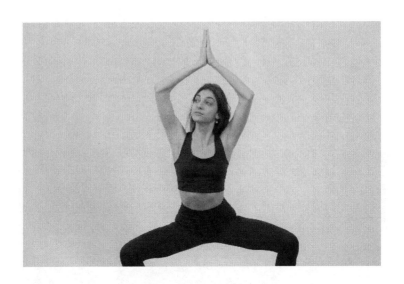

Time:

Depending on your fitness level and preferences, the length of this exercise can change.

It is advised to begin with a lesser time frame, like five to ten minutes, then to progressively extend it as you get stronger and more comfortable.

Materials and equipment required:

Comfortable exercise clothes - Sturdy wall or vertical surface for support - Athletic shoes with adequate traction

Direction

1. With your back to the wall, take a position about two feet away from it.

2. With your toes pointed out at a comfortable angle, place your feet slightly wider than shoulder-width apart.

3. Straighten your arms out in front of you, keeping them parallel to the ground with your palms down. This will support your balance as you perform the activity.

4. Lower your body into a squat stance by slowly bending your knees while maintaining a straight back. Envision sinking into a fictitious chair.

5. Keep lowering your body until your thighs are as close to the floor as it is comfortable for you to be.

Verify that your knees are in line with your toes and do not protrude excessively forward.

6. Take a brief moment to pause at the bottom position and check that your feet are evenly distributing your weight.

7. Straighten your legs and push through your heels to gradually return to the beginning position.

8. Aim for 10 to 15 squats to begin, then repeat the exercise for the required amount of repetitions.

9. To avoid discomfort or overexertion during the workout, take breaks as needed and pay attention to your body.

9.Wall assisted standing forward bend.

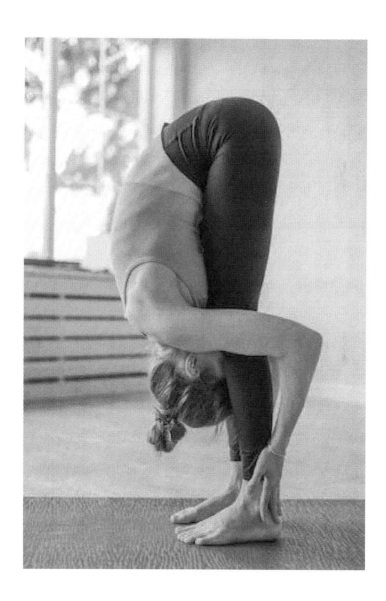

Equipment needed

1. A vertical surface or a strong wall.

Time:

Begin with one or two sets, holding each stretch for fifteen to thirty seconds.
Level 2-3: Hold each stretch for 30-60 seconds in two sets.

Direction

1. Locate an open area next to a wall or other vertical surface.

2. With your feet parallel and hip-width apart, take a stance facing the wall.

3. Step back, approximately an arm's length, from the wall.

4. Line up your shoulders and place both of your hands flat on the wall.

5. To begin, stand up straight and contract your abdominal muscles.

6. Take a deep breath, lengthening your back, and begin the forward bend on the release.

7. Hinge from your hips and descend your body toward your thighs gradually.

8. Keep your legs straight but not locked out. If necessary, keep your knees slightly bent.

9. As you go lower, loosen yourself and let your neck and head drop naturally.

10. Feel a light stretch along the back of your legs as you slowly walk your hands down the wall as far as is comfortable for you.

11. Determine the stretch's depth so that, without going too far, you can feel a slight tension.

12. Breathe slowly and deeply, and attempt to relax and go a little bit further into the pose with each exhale.

13. Maintain a steady breath and a relaxed body while holding this position for the specified amount of time.

14. To come out of the stance, raise your torso, stand tall, and carefully walk your hands up the wall.

15. Take a few seconds to relax and observe how the forward bend affects your body.

10.Wall assisted warrior 111 pose.

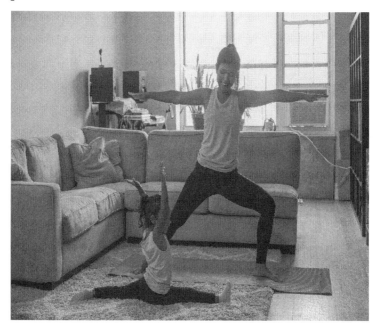

Time Frame:

Depending on your fitness level and preferences, you can choose the length of the workout. As soon as you feel comfortable, start with 1-2 sets of 30 seconds each.

Equipment needed

First, a wall; second, a yoga mat (optional).

Direction

1. Locate a gap in the wall where you can freely extend your arms and legs.

2. Take a position an arm's length away from the wall, facing it.

3. Position your hands shoulder-width apart and at shoulder height on the wall.

4. Point your toes forward and stand tall with your feet together.

5. Inhale deeply, then exhale slowly while slowly raising your right leg straight back and bending your torso forward from the waist. Your right leg should be straight back as you tilt your torso forward and parallel to the floor.

6. For stability and balance, keep your left leg slightly bent.

7. To keep your balance during the posture, contract your core muscles.

8. Pay attention to maintaining a straight line from your hands to your extended back leg while keeping your hips and shoulders pointing toward the floor.

9. To ensure comfort and support, reposition your hand on the wall as necessary.

10. While keeping your breathing constant, hold this position for the required amount of time.

11. Release your lifted leg gradually and return it to its starting position.

12. After taking a brief break, switch to your left leg and repeat the pose.

13. As you get better at your practice, gradually increase the length and quantity of sets.

14. Always pay attention to your body's signals and avoid forcing yourself into a position that hurts or feels unpleasant.

Tips -

Before utilizing a wall as support, make sure it is stable and strong.

- As your strength and balance improve, start with shorter durations and progressively increase.

- Avoid overexerting yourself and instead concentrate on keeping good form and balance.

If you'd want more comfort and support, use a yoga mat or any other type of cushioning material.

10.Wall assisted Chair Pose.

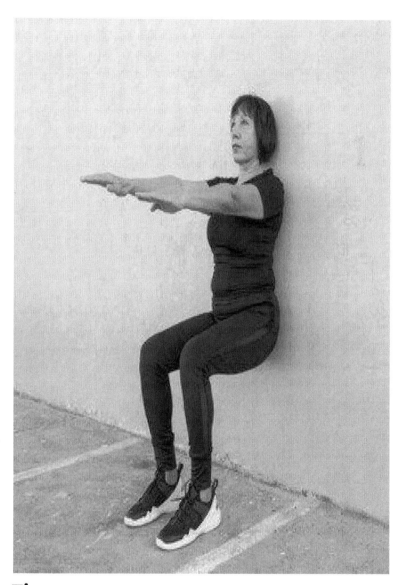

Time:

10 to 15 minutes (warm-up and cool-down included)

Equipment needed

A wall or stable surface

Direction

1. Warm-up: Place your feet hip-width apart and stand upright to begin. Breathe deeply for a few moments, tensing your core and letting your body relax.

2. Locate a wall: Look for an open wall or a stable object that you can rest securely against.

3. Assume a position facing the wall and step back slightly, making sure there's enough room for you to be able to comfortably bend your knees.

4. Align your feet: Set them hip-width apart, parallel to one another. Ensure that they have a strong grip on the earth.

5. Engage your core: To provide stability and support during the exercise, draw your belly button in toward your spine.

6. rest against the wall: With your shoulders relaxed and your spine straight, gently rest your back against the wall. Make sure the wall is in contact with your full back.

7. Bend your knees: As you slowly bring your body down to the floor, imagine yourself reclining in an imaginary chair. Make sure your knees don't go past your toes by keeping them in line with them.

8. Retain the posture: Try to stay in this position for at least 20 to 30 seconds, if possible. Keep your intensity at a level that is both comfortable and demanding.

9. Modify as necessary: Shift your posture closer or further away from the wall if you experience any pain or strain. Pay attention to your body and modify as necessary.

10. Breathe and unwind: Keep taking deep, calm breaths while you hold the pose. Keep your muscles loose and try not to tense up.

11. Repeat: Try to perform the wall-assisted chair stance three to five times, pausing briefly between each time if necessary.

12. Cool-down: After completing the pose, carefully straighten your legs and inhale deeply a few times. Before continuing, give yourself a few moments to unwind and gently stretch any tense muscles.

11.Wall assisted Single deadlift.

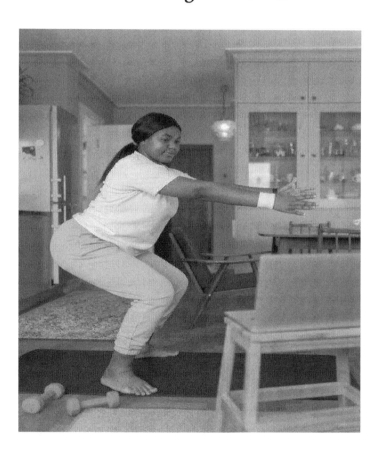

Time

Depending on the number of repetitions you choose and your level of fitness, you can finish this workout in ten to fifteen minutes.

Materials and equipment required:

1. A strong, robust wall
2. Kettlebell or dumbbell (optional)

Direction

1.For this activity, choose an open area close to a solid wall.

2. Take a stand with your back to the wall, making sure you have enough space to completely stretch your arms in front of you.

3. Step into a shoulder-width stance with your toes pointing slightly outward.

4. Raise your arms in front of you so that your hands are flush with the wall at shoulder level.

5. Keep your back straight and engage your core by drawing your belly button toward your spine.

6. Lower your weight gradually onto your right leg while maintaining a flat left foot on the ground.

7. Start the exercise by hunching down and using your glutes to push your hips back, just like you would while shutting a car door. Hold your right knee slightly bent.

8. Keeping your left leg straight behind you and your head in a straight line, elevate it as you tilt forward.

9. Until your torso is parallel to the ground or until your hamstrings feel comfortably stretched, keep bending.

10. Hold this posture for a brief moment, making sure your back is straight and your core is active.

11. Press through your right heel and tighten your glutes to slowly get back to the beginning position.

12. After doing the exercise on the right leg for the required number of repetitions, move on to the left leg.

<u>Tips</u>

Pay close attention to keeping good form the entire time to avoid damage.
If you are unfamiliar with this exercise, begin with a lower weight or just your bodyweight.
Once you're familiar with the exercise, gradually increase the weight or resistance.
- Take a deep breath, release it as you push through your heel to stand.
When holding a dumbbell or kettlebell, make sure it is in the hand opposite the leg you are working on.

12.Wall assisted side leg raises.

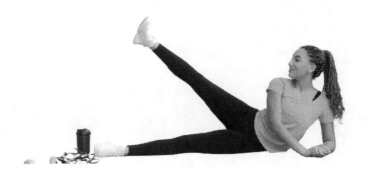

Time:

Ten to twelve repetitions each leg in 1-2 sets can be your starting point. To push yourself, you might progressively increase the amount of sets or repetitions over time.

Equipment required:

a strong, level wall as well as cozy exercise attire and footwear

Direction

1. Place your feet hip-width apart and stand straight, facing a wall.

2. With your arms straight, place your hands on the wall for support.

3. Throughout the exercise, keep your posture upright and activate your core muscles by drawing your belly button toward your spine.

4. Keep your right leg straight and slightly elevated off the ground as you shift your weight to your left leg.

5. Lift your right leg slowly and away from the wall while keeping your balance and control.

6. Raise your leg as high as it will go while maintaining a 45-degree angle with your body.

7. In order to activate your outer thigh muscles, pause a little at the top of the exercise while maintaining your foot flexed.

8. Return your right leg to the beginning position slowly while keeping your balance and composure.

9. On your right leg, perform the exercise for the desired amount of repetitions.

10. To switch sides, put your weight onto your right leg and carry out the same movements as you did with your left.

Tips

 To get the most out of the workout, move slowly and deliberately.
Avoid swinging or depending too much on momentum when lifting your leg laterally; instead, concentrate on engaging your hip muscles.

- Do the exercise in front of a mirror to make sure your leg is raising to the side and to verify your form.
- For extra challenge, if necessary, wrap a resistance band around your ankles.

13.Wall assisted table top.

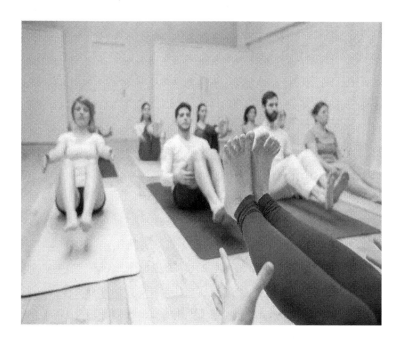

Time:

It normally takes ten to fifteen minutes to finish this exercise.

Equipment needed

1. A clear wall space; 2. An exercise mat or other soft surface (optional).
3. Comfy exercise attire

Direction

1. Locate a clear wall space: Choose a section of a wall where there is no obstacle in your way and you have enough room to complete the activity. Verify that there are no sharp things on the wall and that it is clean.

2. Warm-up: It's crucial to get your body warmed up before beginning an exercise. For a few minutes, raise your heart rate and warm up your muscles by engaging in mild aerobic workouts like jogging, jumping jacks, or brisk walking.

3. Take a position facing the wall: Place your feet hip-width apart and face the wall from a few feet away. Make sure you have adequate room to completely extend your arms.

4. Plant your hands on the wall: Stretch your palms out flat against the wall, slightly wider than shoulder-width apart, at shoulder height. With your fingers pointing upward, that is.

5. Lean forward and raise your legs: Slowly raise your legs off the ground by putting your weight on your hands. Keep your body erect from head to toe by using your core muscles.

6. Hold the posture: Keep your legs raised off the floor and parallel to the ground while maintaining the tabletop posture. Your arms should be at a right angle to your body, which should be slightly slanted. Retain your shoulders away from your ears and your core tightly contracted.

7. Breathe and hold: Maintain the tabletop position while taking calm, deep breaths. As long as you can hold this posture with good form without straining, try to hold it for 20 to 30 seconds.

8. Lower your legs and unwind: Gently return your legs to the floor when you're ready to leave the tabletop posture. Give yourself a chance to unwind and collect your breath.

9. Repeat for desired number of sets: As you gain greater strength and comfort, repeat steps 4–8 for the desired number of sets, progressively extending the length of each set.

10. Cool down: Give your body a few minutes to settle after performing the required number of sets. Take a leisurely stroll and work on your arms, stomach, and legs with some light stretches.

14.Wall assisted supine toe taps.

Time

ten minutes

Equipment includes:

Wall - Exercise mat or towel

Direction

1. To add some padding, find a clean wall space and lay the exercise mat or towel on the ground.

2. Extend your legs straight and place your heels against the wall while lying on your back. With your head and shoulders down on the floor, your torso should make a 90-degree angle with the wall.

3. Pull your belly button gently toward your spine to contract your core muscles. This will assist in keeping your lower back stable during the workout.

4. To start, raise one leg off the wall and extend it as straight as you can toward the ceiling. Throughout the exercise, your other leg should stay in touch with the wall.

5. Keeping your leg straight, slowly lower the raised leg toward the ground. Prior to lifting the leg back up, try to lightly tap your toes on the ground.

6. Try not to jerk or bounce when you tap your toes; instead, concentrate on keeping your movements under control. Continue to move in a controlled, fluid manner.

7. For a predetermined amount of repetitions or for a predetermined amount of time, repeat the toe tap action with the same leg. For each leg, you can begin with 8–10 repetitions, and as you get more comfortable, you can progressively raise that number.

8. Flip over to the second leg and do the same, raising it off the floor, tapping the toes, and lowering it back up again. Throughout, be sure to keep your form and control correct.

9. Keep switching sides for the required amount of time, progressively increasing the length of the workout to ten minutes.

10. Keep in mind to breathe consistently throughout the workout, taking a deep breath before you tap your toes and letting it out as you raise your leg back up.

Tips

Pay attention to your body and only do the activity to the extent that you are comfortable. Avoid forcing yourself to endure pain or discomfort.

See a healthcare provider before performing this activity if you have any prior injuries or medical issues.

To preserve your lower back, always use good form and make sure your core muscles are working.

- Take breaks when necessary, and cease right away if you feel any sudden, intense pain or discomfort.

It is vital to commence with a warm-up and conclude with a cool-down in order to adequately prime and recuperate your body.

You may execute the wall-assisted supine toe taps exercise safely and effectively by following these detailed instructions.

15.Wall assisted glute Bridge.

Equipment needed

A sturdy flat wall

Time:

You can incorporate this activity into your normal fitness regimen for ten to fifteen minutes. Aim for two to three sets of ten to fifteen reps.

Direction

1. Locate a free area up against a wall.

2. Place yourself on your back, knees bent, and feet flat on the floor, about hip-width apart.

3. Assume a close stance against the wall, keeping your feet at arm's length from it.

4. Spread your arms out in front of you, palms down.

5. To establish stability, tuck your lower back into the floor and contract your abdominal muscles.

6. Drive your heels into the wall to start the movement, then drive your hips up toward the ceiling, keeping your knees and shoulders in a straight line.

7. To engage your glutes, or butt muscles, squeeze them at the peak of the exercise.

8. Hold this bridge stance for a little while.

9. Return your hips to the beginning posture gradually, maintaining an engaged gluteal region throughout.

10. Carry out the motion as many times as you like.

Advice: - Keep your knees in alignment with your hips and ankles; avoid letting them droop inward.

Retain a firm core and refrain from arching your back.

Breathe steadily the entire exercise, taking a breath when you descend and a release when you ascend.

 Modify your posture or limit the range of motion if you experience any lower back strain.

16.Wall assisted Forearm plank.

Equipment needed

1. A strong wall

Time frame:

As you gain strength and endurance, start off by holding the position for 20 to 30 seconds, and then progressively extend it.

Direction

1. Locate a spot on a wall that is clear, then face it.

2. With your elbows exactly beneath your shoulders, place your forearms flat against the wall at a distance equal to your shoulders.

3. Take a step backward until you are at a comfortable distance from the wall, keeping your head and heels in a straight line.

4. Place your feet such that your toes are in contact with the wall and they are hip-width apart.

5. Bring your navel toward your spine to activate your core.

6. Maintain a straight posture; do not sag or bend at the hips.

7. Apply pressure by gently pressing your forearms onto the wall.

8. Maintain this posture while breathing steadily throughout the exercise.

9. Pay attention to maintaining your posture and using your core muscles.

10. Re-engage your core and, if needed, modify your technique if you have any lower back pain.

11. Try to stay in this position for as long as you want to or until your form starts to suffer.

12. As your strength increases, progressively extend the duration.

Advice:-If it's difficult for you to keep your form correct, move a step toward the wall.

Stabilize your body by using your thigh and gluteal muscles.

Refrain from lowering your head or shrugging your shoulders.

- Keep in mind to breathe consistently during the activity.

17.Wall assisted dead bug.

Time:

Aim for two to three sets, with ten to fifteen repetitions each. If you're a newbie, start with fewer repetitions and work your way up to a higher number as you gain familiarity.

Equipment needed

A sturdy flat wall

Direction

1. Locate an open wall area first. Assume a facing posture and maintain an arm's length distance from the wall.

2. Raise your arms in front of you and place your palms shoulder-height against the wall. For stability, place your hands shoulder-width apart and spread your fingers widely.

3. Pull your body back into an upright posture by tightening your core and taking a single foot step back.

4. Lift both of your opposing arms and legs at the same time, keeping them parallel to the floor and stretching them straight out in front of you. Keep your core strong the entire time you perform the exercise.

5. Return your arm and leg to the starting position gradually while keeping your balance and steadiness. Try not to overarch your lower back when performing this movement.

6. Raise the second arm and leg at the same time as you repeat the motion on the other side.

7. Keep switching sides, making sure your movements are steady and under control.

8. Keep in mind to breathe consistently during the workout, taking a breath as you elevate your arm and leg and an inhale when you lower them back down.

9. Pay close attention to keeping your technique and control throughout the workout. Movement quality is more significant than movement quantity or speed.

10. As you gain strength and comfort in performing the exercise, gradually increase the number of sets and repetitions.

18.Wall assisted scissors kick.

Equipment needed:

1. A stable wall with adequate room to carry out the exercise securely.

2. Socks or athletic shoes for improved traction (optional).

Time Frame:

Depending on your fitness level and objectives, you can start with two to three sets of ten to twelve repetitions. If necessary, take pauses in between sets.

Direction

1. Locate a free, open wall space. Verify that there are no adjacent risks or things that could impede your movement.

2. Take a stand with your back to the wall and place yourself about an arm's length away from it. Place your feet shoulder-width apart.

3. To provide stability and support, place your hands flat against the wall at shoulder height with your fingers spread wide.

4. With your shoulders slightly over your wrists and your back straight, slant your upper body forward. This is where you will begin.

5. Raise your right leg off the floor and bring it up to your chest, bending the knee.

6. As though you were kicking with force, quickly stretch your right leg forward in a scissor-like action. As far back as you can easily kick your leg without losing your balance.

7. As if you were kicking backward, simultaneously swing your left leg backward in a scissor-like manner. Strive to kick your left leg back as far as you can while keeping it straight.

8. Quickly swap the positions of your legs as your left leg reaches its extension backward and your right leg reaches its extension forward. Your right leg should kick backward, and your left leg should advance.

9. Using the wall for support, repeat the scissor kicking motion, switching up the positions of each leg.

10. Throughout the workout, concentrate on keeping your action smooth and under control. To help regulate the movement and balance your body, contract your core muscles.

11. Perform the activity as prescribed by your fitness regimen or for the appropriate amount of repetitions.

19.Wall assisted oblique V ups.

Time:

You can complete three sets of ten to twelve repetitions on each side of this exercise. The overall duration may change based on how quickly you go and how much you rest.

Equipment needed

1. A wall or other vertically stable surface

2. A cushioned surface or an exercise mat for more comfort (optional)

Direction

1. In your exercise space, locate a clear wall or a strong vertical surface.
2. Take a stance facing the wall and place your feet shoulder-width apart.
3. To provide support, lean against the wall and rest both hands on it.
4. Fully extend your arms, making sure they are straight and fixed in place.
5. Pull your navel in toward your spine to activate your core muscles.
6. Raise your feet just a little bit off the ground while bending your knees slightly and maintaining your legs together.
7. This is where you are going to start.

8. Bending at the waist, slowly elevate your legs toward the right side while maintaining a straight back and arms against the wall. During this motion, you shouldn't move your upper body.

9. Keep rising until your torso and legs are at a 45-degree angle, making a "V" shape.

10. Squeeze your right side oblique muscles at the peak of the exercise.

11. To fully engage the oblique muscles, hold the contraction for a short while.

12. Return your legs to the beginning position slowly, making sure that the action is controlled.

13. On the right side, repeat steps 8–12 as many times as needed.

14. If necessary, take a little break before moving to the left.

15. Carry out steps 8–14 again, but raise your legs to the left this time.

16. To finish a set, perform the required number of repetitions on the left side.

17. To recover, take a 30- to 60-second break in between sets.

Tips

To balance your body and successfully target the oblique muscles, concentrate on maintaining your core engaged throughout the exercise.

Steer clear of using momentum or swinging your legs to complete the exercise. Continue to move deliberately and with control.

- You can do this exercise on the floor with your hands behind you for support if you have trouble maintaining your balance against the wall.

- If you feel any pain or discomfort while exercising, stop right away and get advice from a trained fitness expert.

20.Wall assisted hip hinge.

Equipment needed

1. A strong wall or other vertical object

2. An exercise mat is optional but comfortable.

Time:

five to ten minutes, depending on your objectives and degree of fitness.

Direction

1. Make sure you have enough room and a clear area in front of you before standing erect with your back to the wall.

2. Spread your toes slightly apart and place your feet hip-width apart.

3. Pull your belly button in the direction of your spine to contract your core muscles.

4. With your palms facing down, place your hands on your hip bones. This will act as a point of reference for the duration of the activity.

5. With your shoulders relaxed and your back neutral, slowly bend forward, pushing your hips back towards the wall.

6. Maintain control over the motion by concentrating on bending at the hips rather than the waist. Maintain a balanced weight distribution on both feet.

7. Keep lowering your torso until your hamstrings start to gently stretch. Preventing pain and excessive bending of the spine is crucial.

8. After you've reached your comfortable range of motion, pause briefly. Inhale deeply, then release the breath gradually.

9. To return to the beginning posture, contract your glute muscles and push through your heels while keeping your movement deliberate.

10. Perform the activity as prescribed by your fitness expert or for the appropriate amount of repetitions.

11. Make sure you keep your back straight and your core tight throughout the workout.

12. Keep in mind to breathe regularly and not to hold your breath while performing the exercise.

Tips to Improve Balance and Stability: Begin with a limited range of motion and work your way up as you get more comfortable and flexible; - Use the wall as support if necessary.

To ensure proper form, perform this exercise in front of a mirror or first under the supervision of a fitness professional.

21.Wall assisted clamshells.

Equipment needed

1 A soft surface or exercise mat
- Wall - Resistance band, optional (for increased resistance)

Time Frame:

- For a beginner's session, start with 10 to 15 minutes, and as you get better, progressively extend the time.

Direction

1. Position the exercise mat or other soft surface on the floor in front of a wall in an open area.

2. Make sure your feet are hip-width apart as you stand with your back to the wall.

3. To go into a half squat, slide down the wall with your knees slightly bent. Your knees should be higher than your ankles and your thighs should be parallel to the floor.

4. Pull your belly button in the direction of your spine to contract your core muscles. During the exercise, keep your back flat against the wall.

5. For balance, place your hands on your hips or out in front of you.

6. Lift your right leg slowly away from the wall while maintaining a 90-degree bend in your knee. This is where you are supposed to start.

7. Keep your body in this posture and extend your right knee away from the wall. Envision attempting to elevate the upper leg while maintaining its pressure against the wall to provide resistance.

8. When you notice a slight contraction in your glute muscles, pause for a moment.

9. Bring your leg back to the initial bent position against the wall by slowly bringing your right knee back to the starting position.

10. Perform the required number of repetitions (e.g., 8–12 reps) of this action.

11. Change sides and move your left leg in the same manner.

12. Once you've completed the suggested amount of sets or time, keep switching between the right and left sides.

13. To make the exercise harder, you can, if you'd like, wrap a resistance band around your thighs, just above the knees.

22. Wall assisted donkey kicks.

Time:

Depending on your level of fitness and preferred intensity, you can perform the exercise for ten to fifteen minutes.

Equipment needed

1. A soft surface or exercise mat (optional)
2. A wall or other stable vertical surface

1. Locate a wall or other stable vertical surface that provides ample room to carry out the activity.

2. Take a position facing the wall at a distance of about an arm's length. With your hands slightly

wider than shoulder-width apart, place them on the wall at shoulder height.

3. Place your feet hip-width apart and take a few steps back from the wall. This is where you will begin.

4. Throughout the workout, maintain a straight back and contract your core muscles.

5. To slightly lean your body against the wall and create a tiny angle, bend your knees and lean forward. Stay in this posture for the duration of the workout.

6. Keeping your right leg at a 90-degree angle, raise it off the ground from this starting position. Bend at the knee.

7. Keep your foot flexed and kick your right leg upward, trying to extend it fully. As you extend your leg, tighten your glutes. While you're kicking, release your breath.

8. Concentrate on contracting your glute muscles and keeping your supporting leg stable as you kick upward.

9. At the peak of the exercise, pause for a brief period of time and feel your glutes contract.

10. Bending at the knee, slowly lower your right leg back to the starting position.

11. Switch to your left leg and repeat the motion. For the specified number of repetitions or amount of time, alternate between your right and left leg.

12. Keep your composure and refrain from swinging your legs violently during the workout.

Note: If you experience any pain or discomfort while exercising, stop right away and get advice from a fitness expert.

23.Wall assisted side lunges.

Equipment needed

1. A strong wall or other stable vertical surface is required equipment.

Time
  As you get more accustomed to the workout, you can progressively extend the session from 10 to 15 minutes.

1. Assume an upright position and face the wall with your back to it.

2. Spread your toes forward and place your feet slightly wider than shoulder-width apart.

3. For support, place your hands on the wall in front of you.

4. To keep yourself stable during the workout, contract your core muscles.

5. Move to the left or right, spreading your feet widely enough to make a comfortable lunge possible.

6. As you lower your body into a lunge position on the side where you stepped, bend your hip and knee.

7. Maintain a straight back and make sure your knee and toes are in line.

8. Feel the stretch in your inner thigh as you pause briefly in the lunge position.

9. While maintaining an engaged core, push through your heel to get back to the starting position.

10. For the required number of repetitions, repeat the lunge on the same side.

11. Alternate between the right and left sides while you perform the exercise on the other side.

12. Try to get as many repetitions on each side as you can easily do, ranging from 10 to 15.

13. Focus on good technique and range of motion while moving slowly through the exercise.

14. Unwind and let yourself calm down after doing the required number of sets.

Always pay attention to your body's needs and get advice from a healthcare provider or fitness expert before beginning a new exercise regimen.

24.Wall assisted reverse lunges.

Equipment needed:

1. A stable wall or other vertical surface

Time: As part of a fitness regimen, this exercise can be done for 10 to 15 minutes

Direction

1. Place your feet hip-width apart and face the wall from an arm's length distance to start.

2. With a solid grasp, place your hands at chest height on the wall.

3. Pull your belly button in the direction of your spine to activate your core.

4. Keeping your left foot firmly planted, take a step back with your right foot, allowing your heel to lift off the ground.

5. Keep your torso erect and bend your left leg as you take a step backwards toward the floor.

6. Ensure that your left knee does not extend past your toes as you lower your body until your left thigh is parallel to the ground or slightly lower.

7. After a brief pause, bring your right foot forward to meet your left foot and push through your left heel to get back to the beginning position.

8. Carry out the motion again, taking a step back with your left foot this time.

9. For the required amount of reps or amount of time, switch between your right and left leg.

10. Pay attention to keeping your balance and stability by leaning on the wall during the workout.

11. Avoid hurrying through the workout and maintain control over your movements.

12. Keep in mind to breathe consistently during the activity.

13. You can increase the depth and quantity of your lunge repetitions as you gain comfort and confidence.

Tips:

Before beginning any new workout program, it is always a good idea to speak with a trained fitness instructor or healthcare provider, particularly if you have any pre-existing medical conditions or concerns.

25.Wall assisted curtsy lunges.

Time:
Depending on your fitness level and the amount of repetitions you choose to execute, this exercise should take you between ten and fifteen minutes to finish.

Equipment needed

Sturdy wall or vertical surface - Comfy exercise clothes - Athletic shoes (optional) - Hydration bottle

Direction

1. Choose a good location: Look for a wall or other vertical surface that is free of obstructions and has enough room for you to do out the activity comfortably.

2. Assume a facing position facing the wall, with your arms extended out in front of you. Make sure your feet are hip-width apart, and for stability, tense your core.

3. Adopt good posture: Throughout the workout, maintain a neutral spine, relaxed shoulders, and a straight forward gaze.

4. Place your hands on the wall: Stretch your arms outward so that they are shoulder-width apart, then settle your hands at a comfortable height on the wall. This will give stability and support during the workout.

5. Enter a curtsy lunge: Step your right foot diagonally behind you, crossing it behind and toward your left side of the body. As you bring your body down into a lunge, bend both of your knees to about a 90-degree angle. Your right knee should be slightly off the ground, and your left knee should be precisely over your left ankle.

6. Preserve appropriate form by standing with your hips pointed forward and your weight equally on both legs. Keep your knees from collapsing inward, and make sure your front knee doesn't touch your toes.

7. Push off the wall: To get back to an upright standing position, exhale, press through your left heel, and extend both legs. Throughout this action, maintain your core engaged for stability and control.

8. Switch sides: Carry out steps 5-7 on the other side, placing your left foot diagonally behind you and crossing it over to face your right side.

9. Complete the necessary repetitions: As you build strength and confidence, progressively increase the number of repetitions from the initial few on each side. In the beginning, aim for 8–12 repetitions per leg.

10. Refuel and rest: If necessary, take quick rests in between sets. Drink water to stay hydrated when exercising.

Tips

- If you need more support and stability, put on sports shoes.
- To avoid any abrupt movements and to avoid getting hurt, keep a steady, gradual pace.
- Pay attention to your body and adjust the activity as necessary to fit your fitness level and comfort level.
- If you feel any pain or discomfort during the activity, stop straight away.

26.Wall assisted standing hip abduction.

Equipment needed

A sturdy flat wall

Time frame:

- Warm up your muscles for ten to fifteen minutes at the beginning.

Do two to three sets of ten to twelve repetitions for each leg.

- Take a 30-to 60-second break in between sets.

Directions:

1. Place your feet hip-width apart and stand with your back to the wall.

2. Throughout the exercise, keep your spine neutral and engage your core.

3. For support, place your hands at shoulder height on the wall, little wider than shoulder-width apart.

4. Maintain the straightness of your right leg while shifting your weight to your left leg.

5. Lift your right leg slowly and straight out to the side, as far as is comfortable, from the wall.

6. Avoid twisting your upper body and keep your toes pointed forward.

7. As you reach the end of your range of motion, pause momentarily and feel your outer hip contract.

8. Return your leg to the beginning position with gentleness.

9. Perform the exercise for the required number of times using the same leg.

10. Change sides and work your left leg in the same manner.

Tips

- Instead of depending on momentum or slanting, concentrate on engaging the hip muscles to raise your leg.

- For stability, keep your standing leg slightly bent.

- Try not to slouch or arch your lower back when performing the exercise.

- Begin with a limited range of motion and progressively expand it as your strength and comfort level rise.

- If you experience any pain or discomfort, reduce the amount of movement or consult a fitness expert for advice.

27.Wall assisted standing hip extension.

Equipment needed

A sturdy flat wall

Time:

Perform two to three sets of ten to fifteen repetitions on each leg. Depending on your comfort level and degree of fitness, you can change the quantity of sets and repetitions.

Directions:

1. Place your feet shoulder-width apart and a few inches apart from a sturdy wall while facing it.

2. For support, place your hands slightly wider than your shoulders on the wall at shoulder height.

3. Pull your belly button gently toward your spine to contract your core muscles.

4. Raise your right leg slowly off the ground, stretching it behind you while maintaining its straight posture.

5. Throughout the exercise, keep your left knee slightly bent.

6. Try to maintain your hips parallel to the wall and square. Refrain from moving your hips or tilting your pelvis.

7. Keep extending your right leg backward until your hip flexors begin to gently stretch.

8. Maintain the extended posture for one to two seconds, paying attention to stability and balance.

9. Return your right leg to the beginning position slowly.

10. To complete one repetition, repeat moves 4 through 9 with your left leg.

11. Repeat the required number of times, alternating between the legs.

<u>Tips</u>:

- Make sure you move slowly and deliberately during the workout.

- Pay attention to keeping your back straight and avoiding excessive bending or arching.

- For extra comfort and support, insert an exercise pad underneath your standing foot if necessary.

- As your flexibility increases over time, gradually extend your range of motion.

28.Wall assisted standing knee raises.

Equipment needed

Direction

1. To begin, place your feet shoulder-width apart and face a wall.

2. With your hands slightly wider than shoulder-width apart and at shoulder height, place

them on the wall. Make sure your arms are fully extended.

3. Throughout the workout, keep your posture tall and erect by using your core muscles.

4. Maintain contact with the ground with your left foot while you shift your weight to your right leg.

5. Lift your left foot slowly off the ground while bending and bringing it close to your chest.

6. Keep your back straight and resist the urge to sag forward or backward as you raise your knee.

7. Retain your elevated knee position for a little moment while keeping your balance.

8. Return your left foot to the starting position slowly.

9. Perform the exercise for the required number of times on the same leg.

10. Change your legs and work your right side in the same manner.

Tips: - If you're new to this exercise, start with a reduced range of motion and progressively expand it as you get more at ease.

-Keep the movement moving at a constant, regulated rate.

- You can put your hand on the wall for support and balance if necessary, but as you gain stability, aim to rely less on it.
- To ensure stability during the exercise, concentrate on using your core muscles.

29.Wall assisted standing hamstring curls.

Equipment needed

A sturdy flat wall

Duration:

For each leg, try three sets of ten to fifteen repetitions. Start with a weight and intensity that are difficult for you, but within your reach. Between sets, take a 30- to 60-second break.

Direction

1. Place your feet hip-width apart and face the wall.

2. For support, place your hands shoulder-height on the wall.

3. Throughout the workout, maintain a straight back and engage your core.

4. Raise your right foot off the ground while pushing your heel toward your glutes and flexing your knee.

5. As you raise your foot, contract your hamstrings, or the back of your thigh.

6. Feel the contraction in your hamstrings as you hold the position for a brief period of time.

7. Return your foot to the starting position gradually, keeping it just off the ground to prevent full contact.

8. Complete the necessary number of repetitions with the same exercise on your right leg.

9. Flip to your left leg and carry out the same actions again.

10. Keep in mind to manage your breathing and your movement during the activity.

Tips: - If you have any knee concerns or are new to this exercise, start with a minor bending of the knee.

- Instead of depending too much on momentum or a lot of upper body movement, concentrate on using your hamstrings to lift your foot.

- If you struggle with balance, think about standing on an exercise mat or cushion for increased stability. As your strength and endurance improves, progressively increase the amount of repetitions or sets.

30.Wall assisted standing calf raises.

Equipment needed

A sturdy flat wall

Time frame:

You may start with 2-3 sets of 10-12 repetitions and gradually increase as you become more comfortable with the exercise.

Direction

1. Look for a solid wall or open space where you can stand up straight. For support, place your hands shoulder-width apart on the wall.

2. Place your heels slightly off the floor, toes pointed forward, and feet shoulder-width apart.

3. Pull your belly button toward your spine and maintain a straight posture to activate your core muscles.

4. Push up onto your toes and slowly lift your heels as high as you can. Focus on raising your body weight using your calf muscles.

5. Feel the strain in your calf muscles as you hold the elevated position for a little while.

6. Carefully bring your heels back down to the beginning position.

7. Carry out the exercise as many times as you choose.

8. If necessary, take a little break in between sets before moving on to the next sets.

31.Wall assisted squat with medicine ball.

Time:

Depending on your level of fitness and the amount of repetitions you choose, you can complete this workout in 10 to 15 minutes.

Materials and equipment required:

1. A medicine ball with the proper weight (start light and work your way up)

2. A stable wall or a level, vertical surface

Direction

1. Place your feet hip-width apart and face the wall.

2. Place the medicine ball at chest height and hold it with both hands.

3. Assume a close posture against the wall, keeping your toes pointed slightly outward and your feet comfortably spaced apart.

4. Pull your belly button toward your spine while keeping your back straight to activate your core muscles.

5. Sit back into a squat stance and bend your knees to start lowering your body towards the ground.

6. Keep your back straight, your eyes forward, and your chest up as you lower yourself.

7. Your knees should line up with your toes and your thighs should be parallel to the ground or slightly lower at the lowest point of the squat.

8. Maintain the squat for a short while, then release your breath and drive through your heels to go back to the beginning, completely extending your legs.

9. Complete the required number of repetitions of the squat.

10. Throughout the workout, make sure you stay in control and refrain from bouncing or jerking.

Advice for good form: - Avoid placing most of your weight on your toes and instead distribute it to your heels and midfoot.
- Actively push your knees outward rather than allowing them to collapse inward.
- Throughout the motion, keep your spine in a neutral position.
- As you raise yourself back up, contract your glute muscles.

32.Wall assisted rotational squat.

Equipment needed

A sturdy flat wall

Time frame:

As soon as you feel comfortable with the workout, you can progressively extend the length from 10 to 15 minutes.

Direction

1. Place your feet shoulder-width apart and point your toes slightly outward while facing a firm wall.

2. With your palms flat against the wall in front of you, place your hands on the wall at shoulder height.

3. Throughout the workout, keep your posture straight and contract your core muscles.

4. Lower yourself into a squat slowly, pushing your hips back and bending your knees.

5. When you squat, make sure your knees stay within your toes and maintain a straight back.

6. Take a moment to concentrate on your stability and balance once you've reached the bottom of the squat.

7. Keeping your hands on the wall for support, start rotating your upper body to one side while still squatting.

8. Rotate to the extent that it is comfortable for you, feeling your hips and lower back stretch.

9. After a little period of holding the rotating position, slowly rotate back to the initial position.

10. Straighten your legs and push through your heels to go back to the beginning position.

11. On the opposite side, perform the squat and rotational exercise again.

12. For the required number of repetitions or amount of time, keep switching up the rotations.

33.Wall assisted tuck jumps.

Equipment needed

A sturdy flat wall

Time frame:

Depending on your level of fitness, you can execute this exercise for a set amount of time or repetitions. Aim for two to three sets of ten to twelve repetitions, taking a 30- to 60-second break in between.

Directions:

1. Place your feet shoulder-width apart and face a wall.

2. With your hands at shoulder height on the wall and your arms out in front of you, take a position one to two feet away from the wall. Place your palms flat against the wall.

3. Inhale deeply and be ready to jump.

4. Keeping your back straight and your core active, bend your knees and lower your body into a squat position. Your toes and knees should be parallel.

5. Use both feet to explode off the ground and launch yourself as high as you can.

6. As soon as you can, bring your knees as close to your chest as you can while you're in midair.

7. Return to the beginning squat position by spreading your legs wide again and landing gently.

8. As soon as you touch down, push off the ground once again to get ready for the next repetition.

9. To get the required amount of repetitions or length, repeat steps 4 through 8 again.

Keep in mind to: - Keep your form correct throughout the exercise.

- To steady your body, contract your core muscles.

- For balance and support, use the wall.
- To reduce the force on your joints, land gently.

Gentle Stretches and movement to improve flexibility.

1. Forward Fold Standing:

Place your feet hip-width apart as you stand. Lean forward slowly from the hips, allowing your upper body to drop to the floor. Let your hands fall to your ankles, shins, or the ground. Breathe deeply while holding this stretch for 30 seconds.

2. The Cat-Cow Pose:

With your wrists exactly behind your shoulders and your knees beneath your hips, start out on your hands and knees. Take a deep breath, arch your back, raise your chest to the ceiling, and let your belly drop to the floor (cow posture). Exhale and curve your spine upward, bringing your chin to your chest in the "cat pose." Continue in this manner for eight to ten rounds, breathing as you go.

3. Forward Bend While Seated:

With your legs out in front of you, take a seat on the floor. As you exhale, softly walk your hands forward, folding them at the hips. Inhale and stretch your spine. Take a comfortable reach and hold it for a duration of 30 seconds. In case you have any lower back discomfort, don't forget to maintain a modest bend in your knees.

4. The Butterfly Extend:

Place your feet together so that they are touching while you sit on the floor. Gently press your elbows into your inner thighs to encourage them to open up while holding onto your feet or ankles. Start bending forward from your hips, letting your knees drop to the floor on their own. While taking deep breaths, hold this stretch for 30 seconds.

5. Quad Stretches While Standing:

Put your feet hip-width apart and stand tall. With your right hand, grasp your right foot or ankle while you flex your right knee and bring your right heel up to your glutes. To further extend the stretch at the front of the thigh, softly drive your right hip forward while keeping your balance by engaging your core. After 30 seconds of holding, swap sides.

Breathing for relaxation & stress relief.

Breathing exercises are a particularly useful technique for women going through menopause when it comes to relaxation and stress alleviation.

Significant hormonal changes occur during the menopause, which can cause a range of mental and physical symptoms including mood swings, hot flashes, insomnia, and elevated stress levels. Regularly practicing breathing techniques will help you relax, lower your anxiety, and

and foster a feeling of health. Here, we'll look at five easy-to-learn breathing techniques that are particularly effective for menopausal women.

1. Deep Belly Breathing: Close your eyes while sitting or lying down in a comfortable position. Grasp your abdomen with one hand and your chest with the other.

Inhale deeply through your nose, feeling your abdomen rise as air fills your lungs.

Breathe out slowly through your mouth while you feel your stomach contract.

For many minutes, keep repeating this process while paying attention to how your breath enters and exits your body.

By assisting in the activation of the parasympathetic nervous system, deep belly breathing reduces stress and encourages relaxation.

2. 4-7-8 Breath:

Maintain a straight spine while sitting comfortably.

Shut your eyes and inhale deeply through your nose while silently counting to four.

For seven counts, hold your breath. Breathe out slowly via your mouth while counting to eight.

Do this cycle four or five times. During menopause, the 4-7-8 breath technique can be very helpful as it helps to lower anxiety, heart rate, and relax the nervous system.

3. Alternate Nostril Breathing: Sit upright in a comfortable position. Using your thumb to close your right nostril, take a deep breath through your left nostril.

With your ring finger closed, let go of your thumb, and exhale through your right nostril.

Breathe in via your right nostril, shut it with your thumb, then release the breath through your left nostril.

For five minutes, repeat this cycle while paying attention to how breath enters and exits each nostril.

By balancing the brain's hemispheres, alternate nostril breathing can ease stress and improve mental clarity.

4. Gradual De-stressing Breathe: Close your eyes while sitting or lying down in a comfortable position. To start, inhale deeply, then slowly exhale to release any tension in your body.

Start with your toes, take a deep breath, and squeeze them tightly for a little while. Then let go of the stress by exhaling.

Repeat this procedure for your feet, calves, thighs, belly, chest, arms, and lastly, your face as you slowly work your way up your body.

Deep relaxation can be facilitated by releasing physical and mental stress through the use of gradual muscle relaxation in conjunction with this breathing practice.

5. Counted Breathing: Find a comfortable posture to sit or lie down, then close your eyes. Inhale deeply while silently counting to four.

After holding your breath for four counts, release it for the same number of counts. Take a breath and pause for a further four counts.

For several minutes, keep repeating this process while concentrating on your breathing and the rhythmic counting.

Calm and relaxation are achieved by the regulation of breathing patterns through the practice of counted breathing.

Tips

Including these breathing techniques in your regular practice can help alleviate stress, anxiety, and menopausal symptoms in a big way.

Remember that in order to get the full rewards, consistency is essential. Set aside some time each day, in a place that is comfortable and quiet, to totally immerse yourself in the calming power of your breath.

Chapter5: Targeting Common Menopause symptoms.

Managing hot flashes & night sweats through specific Exercises.

For many people, especially those going through menopause, hot flashes and nocturnal sweats can be upsetting and uncomfortable.

Although physical activity might not totally eradicate these symptoms, including particular activities in your regimen might assist in controlling and lowering the frequency and severity of hot flashes and night sweats. The following workouts could be helpful:

1. Cardiovascular exercises: Regular cardiovascular activity, such as jogging, cycling, swimming, or walking, can help control body temperature and enhance general cardiovascular health. On most days of the week, try to get in at least 30 minutes of moderate-intensity exercise.

2. Yoga: As it encourages relaxation and lowers stress, yoga can be very helpful in controlling hot flashes and night sweats. Some positions might be very beneficial, like inversions, standing poses, and forward bends. To further reduce discomfort, concentrate on deep breathing exercises and relaxation methods.

3. Strength training: Including strength training activities in your regimen will assist lower body fat percentage and build muscle strength, both of which can lessen the frequency of hot flashes and nocturnal sweats. Give special attention to activities that work your huge muscle groups, such weightlifting, squats, lunges, and push-ups.

4. Pelvic floor exercises: Also referred to as Kegel exercises, these exercises assist strengthen the pelvic muscles and enhance control over the bladder. For the treatment of night sweats that may be connected to incontinence, this can be very helpful.

5. Mind-body exercises: Techniques like tai chi and qigong combine deliberate, slow motions with meditation and deep breathing.

These activities may help lessen hot flashes and night sweats by fostering relaxation, lowering stress, and balancing hormone levels.

6. Cooling exercises: Include activities that cause the body to cool down, including water aerobics or swimming.

Engaging in these activities can help control body temperature and alleviate hot flashes and nocturnal sweats.

Never forget to speak with your doctor before beginning a new fitness regimen, particularly if you have any underlying medical issues.

It's important to pay attention to your body and modify the length and intensity of exercises to suit your comfort level.

Wearing breathable clothing, avoiding trigger foods and drinks (such as alcohol, caffeine, and spicy foods), staying hydrated, managing stress with methods like deep breathing or meditation, and maintaining a healthy weight are additional lifestyle changes that may help manage hot flashes and night sweats in addition to exercise.

Exercise can help control hot flashes and night sweats, but it's crucial to have reasonable expectations.

While everyone's experience is unique, some people may need extra help or medication to adequately manage these symptoms.

Strengthening Pelvic Floor Muscles for better bladder Control

For women going through menopause, maintaining bladder control might be a typical issue.

Women may have changes in their pelvic floor muscles at this time, which can impact bladder function as estrogen levels drop.

movements designed to strengthen these muscles, such as wall Pilates movements, can assist improve bladder control and pelvic health in general.

A set of muscles called the pelvic floor supports the rectum, uterus, and bladder.

Pilates exercises, which emphasize stability and strength in the core, are an excellent way to target and build these muscles.

Because they use the wall as resistance and offer a steady platform for support while working on pelvic floor activation, wall Pilates movements are very helpful.

Locate a peaceful area with a blank wall to begin. Put on loose clothing and take a position arm's length away from the wall, facing it. Make sure your back is straight and your feet are hip-width apart. Breathe deeply for a few moments to help you center.

The first workout is referred to as "Wall Squats." Make sure your entire spine touches the wall as you erect yourself and lean your back against it.

As you slowly descend the wall, bend your knees to a ninety-degree angle. Make sure your back is on the wall and your knees are directly above your ankles as you hold this posture for a few seconds.

To get back to standing, slowly push through your heels and contract your pelvic floor muscles.

After ten repetitions, progressively increase the number as you get more familiar with the activity.

An additional useful exercise is the "Wall Bridge." Lay flat on your back with your knees bent, feet pressed up against the wall, and arms by your sides.

Using your pelvic floor muscles, slowly raise your hips off the floor. After a few period of holding this position, return your hips to the floor. For ten repetitions, repeat this exercise, being mindful to keep your pelvic floor engaged.

Furthermore, the "Wall Sit" exercise is quite helpful. Place your feet hip-width apart and lean your back against the wall. Bend your knees and slowly glide down the wall as if you were seated in a chair.

Try to stay in this posture for thirty seconds at a time, and then extend it progressively. Throughout the workout, keep your pelvic floor muscles active.

When it comes to developing the pelvic floor muscles, consistency is essential. Try to include these exercises in your regular routine, and as you become better, progressively up the number of repetitions and length of time.

To avoid pain or strain, it's critical to pay attention to your body and adjust the workouts as necessary.

Better bladder control after menopause can also be attained by leading a healthy lifestyle in addition to Pilates activities.

Remain hydrated, but refrain from consuming too much liquids right before bed or right before working out. Because they can irritate the bladder, avoid or use alcohol and caffeine in moderation.

Use methods for bladder training, such planned voiding, to progressively extend the intervals between bathroom breaks.

Keep in mind that every woman's menopausal experience is different, and it's always best to speak with a healthcare provider before beginning a new exercise program.

Women can improve their general well-being throughout menopause by strengthening their pelvic floor muscles, improving bladder control, and implementing wall Pilates exercises along with the appropriate lifestyle adjustments.

Chapter6: Empowering your Mind: Mindfulness & Meditation

Incorporating mindfulness into wall pilates practice.

I

ncluding attentive elements in your wall Your total experience can be greatly improved and your body and mind can benefit greatly from doing Pilates.

The integration of mindfulness and Pilates concepts can help you develop a stronger connection to your body, enhance focus, lessen stress, and find inner peace.

Let's look at some practical methods for enhancing your wall Pilates practice with mindfulness.

1. Establish an intention: Before starting your wall Pilates exercise, pause to consider what you want to get out of the session.

This could involve establishing balance and self-care, as well as developing strength and flexibility.

By establishing an intention, you give your practice direction and purpose and help you to remain mindful and in the moment.

2. Deep Breathing: One of the most effective ways to focus attention and encourage relaxation is through mindful breathing.

During your wall Pilates exercise, be mindful of your breathing. Breathe in and out slowly and deeply while intentionally contracting your core and bringing your motions into alignment with your breath.

This encourages a calm and concentrated mindset and aids in bringing your attention to the here and now.

3. Body Awareness: Being mindful involves paying attention to your body as well as being totally present in the moment.

As you do wall Pilates, deliberately pay attention to every action and feeling. Observe your body's alignment, the way your muscles contract, and the minute changes in energy.

This increased awareness of your body strengthens the mind-body connection and enables you to move as efficiently as possible.

4. Non-Judgmental Observation: As you work through your wall Pilates movements, try observing your thoughts, feelings, and sensations without passing judgment or feeling any attachment.

Just acknowledge the ideas and let them pass, without categorizing them as pleasant or negative. By encouraging acceptance, this nonjudgmental method lowers stress and improves your capacity for present-moment awareness.

5. Slow Down: It's simple to speed through workouts and ignore the nuances of our motions in our fast-paced lifestyles.

We are reminded to slow down and savor every moment by practicing mindfulness. Whether you're doing a static plank or leg presses against the wall, concentrate on the form of each exercise rather than just getting the job done.

This slow speed improves stability, body control, and ultimately the efficacy of your wall Pilates practice.

6. appreciation Practice: A key component of mindfulness is developing an attitude of appreciation. As you perform your wall Pilates exercise, pause to acknowledge and feel grateful for the tenacity and strength of your body.

Recognize the advantages it offers to your general well-being and the chance to participate in this mindful movement activity.

This small change in viewpoint can greatly improve your mindset and help you develop your mindfulness practice.

Keep in mind that practicing wall Pilates with mindfulness is a journey that takes time and patience.

You will eventually become more conscious in your daily life as well as during your wall Pilates sessions as you continue to practice these strategies.

Thus, seize the chance to combine mindfulness with Pilates and witness the revolutionary impact it can have on your whole mental and physical health.

Techniques for reducing anxiety & improving mental well-being.

For women, Pilates can be a great method to enhance their mental health and lessen worry.

This kind of low-impact, moderate exercise helps to improve balance and soothe the mind in addition to strengthening the body.

We will look at a number of methods in this book that can improve women's Pilates experiences and help them feel better overall.

1. Deep Breathing:

Mindful breathing is one of the core Pilates exercises. Women should be encouraged to concentrate on their breathing by inhaling and exhaling slowly and deeply. By triggering the body's relaxation reaction, this deep breathing method lowers stress and anxiety levels.

2. Mindfulness:

Including mindfulness exercises in your Pilates routine can greatly enhance your mental health.

Urge people to focus on their bodily motions while being aware of their current state of mind and their physical sensations.

Being mindful fosters a focused and peaceful state of mind as well as a stronger feeling of self-awareness.

3. Gentle Stretching:
Pilates entails extending and stretching the muscles gently, which can soothe stress and lessen anxiety.

Women should be encouraged to mindfully perform these stretches so that their bodies can unwind and rest.

Stress the value of paying attention to their bodies and not pushing themselves too much.

4. Setting Intentions: Invite women to make positive self-intentions at the start of each Pilates class.

These goals may have to do with reducing stress, increasing confidence, or enhancing mental health in general.

By establishing goals, people develop drive and a sense of purpose, which improves the experience as a whole.

5. Progressive Muscle Relaxation: Including Pilates-style progressive muscle relaxation exercises can help significantly lower anxiety levels.

People should be taught to contract and then release certain muscle groups in a methodical manner, working their way up to the neck and face from the toes.

This method can ease tension and anxiety and promote profound relaxation.

6. Visualization: During Pilates lessons, lead participants in visualization exercises.

Urge them to visualize oneself in a calm and pleasant setting, like a lovely beach or a peaceful garden.

By refocusing attention from stressors, visualization promotes serenity and peace.

7. Use of Positive Affirmations: Include Pilates workouts with the use of positive affirmations.

To help women reinforce good thoughts and beliefs about themselves, encourage them to repeat affirmations aloud or silently.

This exercise can lessen anxiety, elevate mood, and boost self-confidence.

8. Social Connection: Assist ladies in finding a workout partner or enrolling in group Pilates courses.

Developing relationships with people who have similar interests to yours might lessen feelings of loneliness and enhance mental health.

In addition to fostering a feeling of community, social interaction in Pilates courses can improve motivation and accountability.

9. thankfulness Practice:

Include movements in Pilates classes that focus on thankfulness. Encourage participants to think about three things for which they are thankful before or after each session.

Practicing gratitude lowers anxiety levels, increases feelings of happiness, and improves general well being.

10. attentive Transitions: Instruct women in making attentive movements between Pilates routines. Stress the value of staying in the present and transitioning between movements with elegance. This focused approach lessens distractions, enhances mental clarity, and fosters a general sense of calm.

Women can greatly lower their anxiety levels, enhance their entire experience, and improve their mental health by implementing these tactics into their Pilates practice.

Recall that it's critical to pay attention to your body, move at your own speed, and get advice from a certified Pilates teacher. Savor the process of self-exploration while benefiting from Pilates's mental and physical advantages.

Chapter7: Advance Wall Pilates for Progression.

Challenging Exercises to further enhance strength & stability

1.Wall plank.

Time Frame: Approximately 10-15 minutes

Equipment/ Materials Needed:
1. A sturdy wall
2. Exercise mat or towel (optional)

Direction

1. Choose an appropriate wall: In your exercise area, look for a level, reliable wall.

2. Prepare the wall: Remove any objects or obstructions to make the space secure for exercise.

3. Assume a facing position with your arms extended straight out in front of you.

4. **Foot placement:** Make sure your feet are firmly planted on the ground by spacing them hip-width apart.

5. **Modify the position of your hands:** Lift your arms and reach forward, pressing your palms flat against the wall.

6. **Engage your core:** To stabilize your body, contract the muscles in your abdomen.

7. **Lean forward:** Start by bending forward and, while keeping your torso straight, progressively walk your hands along the wall.

8. **Full plank position:** Hold this position until your arms are fully extended, shoulders are stacked over your wrists, and your torso is parallel to the ground.

9. Length of hold: Maintain this posture for the chosen amount of time. Start out with a goal of 20–30 seconds, and as you become better, progressively extend it.

10. Keep your body in good alignment: Avoid drooping or arching your back by keeping your body straight.

11. Breathe: Throughout the exercise, keep your breathing steady and under control.

12. Release the plank: Gently walk your hands back up the wall until you are standing in order to finish the wall plank.

13. Rest and repeat: After a little break, perform the exercise again for as many sets as you'd like.

<u>Tips</u>

If you are having trouble maintaining proper form, lessen the time or change how you are standing (for example, begin with an inclined wall plank).

If the wall is uneven or uncomfortable, cushion your palms with a towel or an exercise mat.

2.Wall push ups:

Equipment or material needed for this exercise

~sturdy wall~

Time frame

The duration of this exercise might vary depending on your fitness level and goals because you can complete it at your own pace.

As you advance, progressively increase the number of repetitions or duration from the comfortable starting point.

Direction

1. Take a position facing a solid wall that is about an arm's length away.
2. To provide stability, spread your feet shoulder-width apart.
3. Spread your arms out and lay your palms flat, little wider than shoulder-width apart, on the wall at shoulder height.
4. Make sure your core is active and your body is in alignment. A straight line should be formed by your head, shoulders, hips, and heels.
5. Inhale, bending your elbows and lowering your chest gradually toward the wall. Maintain a straight body throughout the exercise.
6. Try to bring your chest down to a mere few inches from the wall. This is where you're going to start.

7. Straighten your arms and push against the wall while exhaling to get back to the beginning position.

8. Carry out the motion for the required number of times or amount of time.

9. Throughout the activity, pay attention to your body and take breaks as needed.

10. You can progressively increase the duration or number of repetitions as you get better and more at ease.

3.Wall squat.

Equipment needed:

A sturdy, flat wall with enough space , comfortable exercise clothing & athletic shoes

Time frame

Start with 3 sets of 10-15 repetitions & gradually increase as you become more comfortable with exercises.

Directions:

1. Place your feet shoulder-width apart while standing with your back to the wall.
2. As you lower your body into a squatting position, slowly slide your back down the wall. Ideally, your knees should be 90 degrees from the body, as though you were sitting in a chair.
3. To guarantee that your weight is distributed equally, keep your feet flat on the ground.
4. Throughout the workout, keep your stability and correct form by using your core muscles.
5. Remain in the squat position for a brief period of time, keeping your back to the wall and your posture correct.
6. To go back to starting position, slowly push through your heels and straighten your legs.
7. After a brief period of rest, perform the exercise again for the required amount of repetitions.

8. Keep in mind to breathe consistently while performing the exercise, taking breaths when you squat and exhale.

Advice to Reduce strain on your knee joints: - When squatting, make sure your knees do not cross over your toes.
- Pay more attention to form and control than to repetition count or pace.
- Be mindful of any pain or discomfort. In the event that you encounter any, stop exercising and seek medical advice.

Wall squats are an excellent lower-body strength training exercise that works the glutes and quadriceps in particular. You can increase your strength and endurance by progressively increasing the amount of sets and repetitions over time. As usual, pay attention to your body's signals and stop if you feel any sudden, intense pain or discomfort.

4.Wall assisted leg Squat.

Equipment needed:
A sturdy flat wall

Time frame:
The variation of the exercise can varies depending on your fitness level and goals,
Start with 2 - 3 sets of 10 repetitions, and gradually increase as you get stronger

Directions:

1. Place your feet shoulder-width apart and face the wall.

2. Depending on how comfortable you are, place yourself one to two feet away from the wall.

3. Maintaining a straight back, place your palms flat against the wall at chest height and slant your body slightly forward.

4. Pull your belly button in toward your spine to activate your core muscles.

5. Take a deep breath and slowly lower your hips toward the floor, as though you were reclining in an imaginary chair.

6. To safeguard your joints, maintain your knees in line with your toes and your weight on your heels.

7. As low as your flexibility will allow, squat down until your thighs are roughly parallel to the floor. Avoid moving past what is comfortable for you.

8. To return to the starting posture, completely extend your hips and knees by exhaling and pushing through your heels.

9. Carry out the motion for the required number of times.

10. You are welcome to use your hands against the wall for stability during the exercise if you require any extra help.

Tips

 Preserve good posture by avoiding rounding your shoulders and maintaining a straight back.

- Take a breath before falling and release it as you push upward to regulate your breathing.

- Instead of depending on your arms or the wall for support, concentrate on using your leg muscles to propel through the exercise.

- As you get more comfortable and flexible, progressively deepen your squat from a shallow starting point.

5.Wall Sit.

Equipment needed:

A sturdy flat wall and a comfortable workout clothes and closed toe shoe

Time frame:

Start with a goal of holding the wall sit position for 30 seconds and gradually increase the time as you become more comfortable and stronger, aim to work up to 1-2 minutes.

<u>Directions:</u>

1. Locate a free wall or level area, then place your back against it.

2. Place your feet about two feet away from the wall, shoulder-width apart.

3. Bend your knees and slowly slide your back down the wall, supposing that you are seated in a chair.

4. Keep sliding down until you reach a comfortable 90-degree angle, or as close to it as possible, with your knees bent. The thighs ought to be parallel to the floor.

5. Make sure your feet are flat and your heels are on the floor; avoid lifting your toes.

6. Maintain a flat back against the wall and pull your belly button in the direction of your spine to contract your core muscles.

7. Rest your arms at your sides or place your hands on your hips.

8. Maintain appropriate form and hold this posture for the specified amount of time. Keep your breathing steady the entire time.

9. When you're ready to stop, effortlessly raise yourself back up with your legs to stand again.

It's crucial to keep the right form throughout the exercise. Refrain from bending forward or letting your knees cross your toes.

- Stop the workout and see a healthcare provider if you feel any pain or discomfort while doing it.

- To prevent overdoing it or getting hurt, gradually increase the amount of time and intensity you spend exercising as you get more comfortable.

6.Wall assisted pike push ups.

Equipment needed:

A sturdy flat wall, & comfortable workout clothes for exercise

Time frame:

It's recommended to perform 2-3 sets of 10-15 repetitions, depending on your fitness level & ability.Rest for about 30 to 60 seconds between sets.

<u>Direction</u>

1. Face a sturdy wall and place your feet hip-width apart. Make sure you have enough space to spread your arms out fully.

2. Spread your hands slightly wider than shoulder-width apart and set them on the wall, fingers pointing upward.

3. Step back from the wall a few feet, keeping your arms outstretched and your posture upright. This is the appropriate place for you to begin.

4. Tense your core and carefully walk your feet up the wall to raise your hips toward the sky. Keep your arms straight at all times.

5. Continue walking your feet up the wall until your body forms an inverted "V" with your hips at the top.

6. Once you're in the pike position, lower your head toward the wall, bend your elbows, and lower your upper body between your hands. Maintain a straight back and an engaged core.

7. Pause for a moment when your head is almost against the wall, then extend your elbows by pushing through your hands and return one step to the starting position.

8. To obtain the desired amount of repetitions, go back and repeat steps 6 and 7.

Tips

-Always do the exercise using proper form. Keep your core active to prevent hunching your hips or arching your back.

- Keep an eye out for intentional movements and a gradual, even decline. Don't use momentum when completing the workout.

- Use an exercise mat or towel to put your hands and feet up against the wall if you have difficulties maintaining your balance.

7.Wall assisted L sit

Equipment needed:

A sturdy flat wall, comfortable workout clothes and a shoe suitable for workout.

Time frame:

Start with a shorter duration, around 10-15 seconds & gradually aim to increase to 30 seconds or more as you build strength and balance.

Directions:

1. Locate a free wall area. Make sure there is adequate space around you so that you can complete the activity safely.
2. Take a position facing the wall that is approximately an arm's length away.
3. Press your hands against the floor with your fingers pointed in the direction of the wall, placing them shoulder-width apart.
4. Bend forward, raise your legs off the floor, and progressively ascend the wall. Maintain an L-shaped body alignment and stretch your legs while you walk.
5. Keep moving up the wall until your torso and legs are at a 90-degree angle and your body is parallel to the ground.
6. Maintain this posture while using your core muscles to provide body stability. Pay close attention to keeping your back straight and your legs parallel to the floor.
7. Hold the pose for ten to fifteen seconds, starting at a time that feels comfortable.

8. As you advance and strengthen your upper body and core, progressively extend the duration.

Tips: - To avoid getting hurt, warm up your body before doing this workout.
- Maintain a comfortable posture with your shoulders down and away from your ears.
- To stabilize your body during the workout, contract your core muscles.
- If you have trouble maintaining your balance at first, work on it by practicing with one foot on the ground until you have the strength and stability needed to raise your legs fully.
- Pay attention to your body and avoid pushing yourself past what is comfortable. Gradually extend the duration over time.

Always remember to check that an exercise program is appropriate for your physical condition by speaking with a healthcare provider or fitness instructor before beginning or altering one.

8.Wall Bridge.

Equipment needed

A sturdy flat wall

Time:

10-15 minutes

Direction

1. In a roomy location, locate a wall or other suitable vertical surface.
2. Make sure there is enough room around you while you stand facing the wall.
3. Position your feet slightly away from the wall, shoulder-width apart.
4. Lift your arms out in front of you and hold them parallel to the floor.
5. Inhale deeply while contracting your abdominal muscles.

6. Lower your hips to the floor and bend your knees as you begin to squat slowly.

7. Lean your back against the wall as you lower yourself into a squat.

8. Make sure your knees are at a 90-degree angle with your ankles.

9. As long as it is comfortable for you, hold this position for ten to fifteen seconds.

10. Throughout the workout, breathe steadily and with proper posture.

11. Press your feet into the ground and raise yourself back up to a standing posture to exit the pose.

12. Complete ten to fifteen repetitions of the exercise, or as many as you choose.

Tips

 - If you experience any pain or discomfort while exercising, stop and see a doctor.

- Throughout the bridge, keep your back straight against the wall to preserve good form and prevent stressing your lower back.
- To support and stabilize your back, concentrate on using your core muscles

9.Wall Assisted Handstand.

Equipment needed

An open wall space with enough space.

Time:

The duration of the exercise can vary depending on your fitness level, but start with short intervals of 10-15 seconds & increase as you progress.

Direction

1. Locate a free wall space that allows adequate room for your body to securely carry out the workout.

2. If you'd like more cushioning and traction, lay a non-slip yoga mat down on the ground.

3. Take a position an arm's length away from the wall, with your back to it.

4. Plant your hands on the ground directly in front of your feet, keeping them firmly planted and shoulder-width apart.

5. Draw your navel inward toward your spine to contract your core muscles.

6. With control, raise your legs and bend forward from the hips in the direction of the wall. Try to touch the wall with both of your feet.

7. Walk your feet up the wall and gradually straighten your body into an upright position by using the wall as support.

8. Maintain a solid shoulder girdle, wrist alignment with shoulders, and arms.

9. To keep your balance and stability, use your leg and core muscles.

10. Keep your head neutral and gaze either directly ahead or slightly down.

11. Take calm, deep breaths while paying attention to your balance.

12. To descend, carefully drag your feet back down the wall until they touch the ground.

13. Take a brief break before trying to perform the exercise again.

Always pay attention to your body's signals and move at your own speed. To guarantee safety, it is advised that you have someone spot you or oversee your practice if you are a beginner.

Before doing this activity, please see a fitness expert or trainer if you have any underlying medical ailments or concerns.

10.Wall Assisted Side plank.

Equipment:

A sturdy flat wall, also a yoga mat or exercise mat (optional)

1: Beginning Position: Place your feet shoulder-width apart and stand close to the wall.
- Place your elbow exactly under your shoulder as you place your forearm against the wall.
Keep your legs together as you extend them.

Step 2: Execution - Make a straight line from your head to your heels by engaging your core and lifting your hips off the ground.
- Breathe in and maintain the pose for a predetermined period of time (start with 20 seconds and increase as your strength allows).

- Maintain a steady posture and refrain from bending or twisting too much.
- Pay attention to keeping your ankle, hip, and shoulder in a straight line and preserving appropriate alignment.

3.Changing Sides - Lower your hips gradually back to the floor after maintaining the pose for the required amount of time.
- Take a few moments to rest before switching sides and going to the other side of the wall.
- Using the same procedures, repeat the practice on the opposite side.

Step 4: Repeat and Advance - Try to complete two to three sets of the wall-aided side plank on each side.
- You can extend the hold time or number of sets as you become more stable and strong.
- Additionally, you can add variations like elevating the upper leg or adding tiny leg lifts.

Modification & variation for different Fitness Levels.

This book will discuss the benefits of wall pilates for women of different fitness levels, as well as modification and variation approaches to take into consideration.

For beginners

Beginning with wall pilates is a great' option if you're new to pilates or haven't exercised regularly. It provides support and stability while letting you progressively increase your strength and flexibility. Here are some beginner-friendly modifications:

1. Wall Squats: Lean against the wall with your back to it and squat down, making sure your knees stay in line with your ankles. After a short while, hold the pose and repeat. Your leg muscles will get stronger with this exercise, which want to strain your joints.

2. Wall Push-Ups: Assume a facing position and place your palms at chest height on the wall. Bending your elbows, lower your body against the wall. Then, push away to regain your starting position. This modified push-up is beneficial for strengthening the upper body.

3. Wall Bridges: Bend your knees while lying on your back with your feet up against the wall. In order to form a bridge position, raise your hips off the ground and then lower yourself back down. Your core muscles and glutes will benefit from this exercise.

For Intermediate Level: To improve your wall pilates program, move on to more difficult exercises once you have developed strength and confidence. You may up the ante on your workout with these variations:

1. Wall Planks: Place your hands on the floor beneath your shoulders and begin in a plank posture with your feet up against the wall. Keep your body in a straight line from your head to your heels to strengthen your upper body and engage your core.

2. Wall Lunges: With your back to the wall, raise your body and face away from it. Keeping your back leg near to the floor, bend your front knee and lunge forward. This workout works your glutes, hamstrings, and quads.

The third exercise is called a wall roll-down. Assume a standing position with your back to the wall. Carefully roll down each vertebrae one at a time until your head, shoulders, and back are flat against the wall. Then, roll back up to a standing position using your core strength. This exercise tones the core and improves spine flexibility.

For Advanced degree: Wall pilates can be an energizing and difficult workout for ladies who have a high degree of fitness and pilates experience. These more complex versions will strengthen your entire body and work several different muscle groups:

1. Wall Handstands: With your back to the wall, stand with your hands shoulder-width apart on the ground. Raise your legs into a handstand and lean against the wall for stability. Balance and upper body strength are enhanced by this workout.

2. Wall Ball Squats: Lean against the wall while holding a medicine ball or weighted ball in front of your chest. Keeping the ball close to your body, lower yourself into a squat position. This sophisticated tweak ups the resistance, making the leg and core workout more intense.

3. Wall Side Planks: Start with your body in a straight line, one arm on the floor, and your feet pressed on the wall. Repeat on the other side after holding this position for a predetermined period of time. This version tests stability and goes for the obliques.

It's important to remember to seek advice from a qualified fitness expert or pilates instructor to make sure you're performing each exercise correctly. To get the most out of wall pilates, be consistent, pay attention to your body, and work your way up through the various fitness levels gradually.

Chapter8: Cool Down & Relaxation.

1. Rolling down the wall:

Step 1: Place your feet hip-distance apart and stand with your back to the wall.

Step 2: Stretch your back and, with your head pressed against the wall, begin to carefully roll down each vertebrae one at a time.

Step 3: Roll back up to the beginning position after pausing briefly once your torso is parallel to the floor.

Step 4: Repeat this motion five to eight times, emphasizing deep breathing and fluid, controlled movements.

2. Wall Shoulder Stretch:

Step 1: Assume a facing position, keeping a gap of arm's length between yourself and the wall.

Step 2: With your fingers pointing upward, place your hands on the wall at shoulder height and a little wider than shoulder-width apart.

Step 3: As you feel a slight stretch in your shoulders and chest, bend forward and let your chest get closer to the wall.

Step 4: Breathe deeply and hold this stretch for 20 to 30 seconds.

Step 5: Repeat two or three times, then slowly release the strain.

3. Wall Calf Stretch:

Step 1: Lean one leg back while maintaining the heel flat on the ground while facing the wall.

Step 2: For support, place both hands at shoulder height on the wall.

Step 3: Feel the stretch in your calf muscle as you lean your body weight forward while maintaining the straight back leg.

Step 4: Repeat the stretch two to three times for each leg, holding it for 20 to 30 seconds before switching sides.

4. Wall Chest Opener:

Step 1: Place your right side against a wall while standing next to it.

Step 2: Raise your right arm to the side, with your elbow slightly bent and your palm shoulder-height against the wall.

Step 3: Feel the stretch in your shoulder and chest as you slowly turn your body away from the wall.

Step 4: Hold the stretch for 20 to 30 seconds, then alternately repeat the motion 2-3 times on the other side.

5. Wall Squats:

Step 1: Place your feet hip-distance apart and stand with your back to the wall.

Step 2: Bend your knees and lower your body into a seated position, as if you were sitting on an imaginary chair, as you slowly slide your back down the wall.

Step 3: Make sure your knees do not go past your toes and try to keep your thighs parallel to the floor.

Step 4: While tensing your core and taking deep breaths, hold this position for fifteen to twenty seconds.

Step 5: To stand back up, slowly press through your heels eight to ten times.

Always pay attention to your body and adjust the exercises accordingly. Before completing the exercises, please see a healthcare provider if you are in any pain or discomfort.

Importance of post workout cool down for Menopausal Women

For menopausal women, cool-down exercises are essential and can improve their general health.

Please pay a close attention down below

1. Lowers the Risk of Injury: The body progressively shifts from an exerted to a resting condition when you cool down after activity.

Your blood pressure and heart rate can gradually return to normal as a result of this procedure.

Menopausal women are more likely to sustain musculoskeletal injuries as a result of altered hormone levels, reduced bone density, and decreased flexibility.

A well performed cool-down can help avoid sprains, strains, and joint pain.

2. Promotes Better Recovery: Excessive exercise can lead to muscle soreness and the buildup of waste products from metabolism, such lactic acid, in the body.

Both increasing blood circulation and eliminating these waste products require a cool-down after an exercise.

Because of the increased blood flow, the muscles receive more oxygen and nutrients, which speeds up their recovery and lessens pain after exercise.

Menopausal women may experience a sped up healing period, which enables them to continue regular workout routines.

3. Controls Body Temperature: Menopausal women frequently have hot flashes and nocturnal sweats. Exercise that is too intense can make these sensations worse.

After exercise, a cool-down phase can assist control body temperature and lessen the severity and frequency of hot flashes.

Women can get relief from extreme discomfort and still reap the advantages of exercise by progressively lowering their body's core temperature.

4. Encourages Calm and Mental Health: Mood fluctuations, nervousness, and trouble falling asleep are some of the effects of menopause.

Deep breathing techniques and mild stretching can be used as part of a post-workout cool-down to enhance mental clarity and relaxation.

The "feel-good" hormones called endorphins are released as a result of these activities, and they have the potential to reduce mood disorders and enhance emotional equilibrium in general.

Menopausal women can lower stress and improve their mental health by implementing a cool-down practice.

5. Preserves Flexibility and Joint Health: Hormonal changes during menopause may cause a reduction in joint suppleness and flexibility.

Stretching exercises, in particular, are essential for preserving flexibility and avoiding joint stiffness during cool-down.

Stretching activities can help menopausal women with greater joint mobility, less pain, and a lower chance of developing age-related conditions including osteoporosis and arthritis. They can also help them relax.

6. Encourages Mindful Reflection: For many women, menopause is a time of transition and introspection. It can be very helpful to use the cool-down period following an exercise as a time for introspection and self-awareness.

You may encourage mindfulness and self-connection by paying attention to your breathing and being in the present moment.

During the menopausal transition, this period of introspection can improve mental clarity, increase self-esteem, and promote personal growth.

In conclusion, the cool-down after a workout is not only a nice-to-have, but a crucial part of an all-encompassing fitness regimen, especially for women going through menopause. Women can lower their risk of injury, improve healing, control body temperature, encourage relaxation, preserve flexibility, and enable focused reflection by adding a cool-down session to their exercise routine. Accepting the advantages of cooling down after exercise can improve menopausal women's general health and quality of life. Women who prioritize their cool-down will be better equipped to face the changing menopausal journey with vigor, strength, and perseverance.

Conclusion.

We have looked at a thorough manual in "Wall Pilates for Menopausal Women," which is designed to specifically address the requirements of ladies going through menopause.

We have given women the tools to effectively manage their menopause symptoms by educating them about the value of exercising during this period of life, offering interactive exercises, and presenting factual information throughout this book.

For women, menopause is a normal transition that results in a variety of emotional and physical changes.

We have clarified the importance of exercise, specifically Wall Pilates, in reducing menopause-related symptoms by comprehending the particular difficulties encountered during this time.

It's clear from our research that Wall Pilates is the best type of exercise for women going through menopause.

Utilizing the wall as a support structure improves stability, balance, and focused muscular activation.

In addition, Wall Pilates' soft and deliberate movements enhance general health, strength, and flexibility.

We have illuminated the significance of exercise in preserving bone density, lowering the risk of osteoporosis, and controlling weight gain by exploring the physiological changes that take place during menopause. Additionally,

Wall Pilates has been shown to offset the aging-related loss of muscular mass and strength, enhance mood by producing endorphins, and enhance the quality of sleep.

Apart from its health advantages, Wall Pilates for menopausal women provides an informative element that enables readers to gain awareness about their bodies and the changes they are going through. We have addressed common menopause symptoms including joint pain, mood swings, and hot flashes and offered enlightening explanations and useful advice to help women deal with these difficulties. Our participatory approach will help readers become conscious of their own journeys towards physical and mental well-being, as well as active participants in those journeys.

This book's activities are specifically designed to address the concerns that menopausal women have in mind. Every exercise comes with comprehensive guidelines, photos, and adjustments to guarantee both safety and customization to suit individual requirements. We encourage an environment of experimentation and discovery by including readers in interactive routines, enabling women to find what works best for them.

This book also stresses the value of stress reduction, healthy eating, and self-care in order to help readers maintain a holistic approach to health. Menopausal women can increase their general vigor and resilience and improve the effectiveness of Wall Pilates exercises by incorporating these factors into their daily life.

We hope that "Wall Pilates for Menopausal Women" will be a dependable tool and a friend for women as they move through this life-changing stage. We want to give our readers the tools they need to take charge of their menopause experience by offering accurate information, thought-provoking analysis, and engaging activities. With the help of Wall Pilates and the information in this book, women may thrive during the menopausal years, accept their changing bodies, and manage their symptoms.

Keep in mind that going through menopause is a special and empowering experience. Women can continue to live life to the fullest, full of strength and joy, by following the advice provided in this book.

<u>Bonus</u>

Recipes to enhance your wall pilates journey.

Starting at a wall The Pilates journey includes both physical practice and careful consideration of appropriate diet.

Eating a balanced, nutrient-rich diet is crucial for optimizing performance and facilitating effective recovery.

We will be sharing a number of recipes in this book that are specially designed to improve your wall Pilates experience.

These recipes are made to provide you the energy you need, encourage the growth and regeneration of your muscles, and improve your general health.

Let's explore these tasty and nutritious food options!

1. Energizing Pre-Workout Smoothie Bowl: To boost energy and improve attention, start your wall Pilates practice with an energizing smoothie bowl full of nutrients. Blend together frozen berries, a spoonful of chia seeds, spinach, almond milk, and a ripe banana. Add granola, sliced fresh fruit, and a drizzle of honey over top for some sweetness.

2. Turmeric Quinoa Salad: This vibrant and nourishing quinoa salad will help your body recover from your workout. As directed on the package, prepare the quinoa and allow it to cool. Combine it with feta cheese, cherry tomatoes, bell peppers, sliced cucumbers, and fresh basil. Toss the salad with a good pinch of turmeric, lemon juice, and olive oil. Turmeric's well-known anti-inflammatory qualities make it an ideal supplement for aiding in muscle recuperation.

3. Baked Salmon with Quinoa and Steamed Broccoli: This high-protein supper choice promotes both muscle growth and repair. Drizzle a fresh salmon filet with olive oil, lemon juice, and herbs. Bake for 15 to 20 minutes, or until thoroughly done. For a hearty and filling supper, serve the salmon over a bed of cooked quinoa and steamed broccoli.

4. <u>Sweet Potato and Chickpea Curry:</u> Savor this aromatic curry that's full of complex carbohydrates and plant-based proteins. Diced sweet potatoes, onion, garlic, and ginger should be sautéed until softened in a big pot. Stir in curry paste, coconut milk, and canned chickpeas. Simmer until the flavors have combined and the potatoes are soft. Serve with quinoa or brown rice for a delicious and filling supper alternative.

5. <u>Recovery Smoothie with Tart Cherry Juice:</u> This reviving smoothie helps muscles recuperate from strenuous wall Pilates exercises. Put almond milk, ripe banana, spinach, a scoop of protein powder, and tart cherry juice in a blender. It has been demonstrated that tart cherry juice lowers inflammation and speeds up healing. Enjoy after blending till smooth!

In conclusion, eating a healthy diet is essential to bolstering your wall Pilates endeavor. These dishes include a wide variety of nutrients, such as carbohydrates for energy, protein for muscle repair, and several vitamins and minerals for general health. Recall that frequent wall Pilates practice combined with a balanced diet will help you reach your fitness objectives and improve your experience in general. Cheers to cooking and having fun on your way to transforming wall Pilates!

Made in the USA
Las Vegas, NV
20 September 2024

95536127R20152